## ADVANCE



"A delightful and wonderfully readable r... attitudes, remarkable personal stories, and practical guidance for the ... become more attuned to the sacred dance of life."
—BARNABY B. BARRATT, PHD, DHS, Director, Center for Tantric Spirituality

"In a stunning tour de force, Carla Tara has embodied the spirit of Tantra, weaving myth, tantric practice, and Argentine tango into an irresistible dance of words and ideas. Her tapestry weaves between her childhood in rural Italy, the sensuality of Tango as Tantra, and a unique and startling revelation of Eve as the archetype of the powerful, fully-embodied woman. This is luscious, feminine writing at its best." —MAEVE FRY, Writer and Opera Singer

"A homeopathic remedy for the hopeless romantic in each of us, Carla's stories show the remarkable capacity of the human heart to grow through adversity and bless the world with wisdom. Read it and weep for here human foibles turn into heroic moments where passion and compassion cause our pain to combust and lift us out of the mundane into the radiance of our true nature, grounded in humble joy." —GERALYN GENDREAU, MS, MFT, co-author and editor, *The Marriage of Sex and Spirit: Relationship at the Heart of Conscious Evolution*, Best Health / Sexuality Book, 2006 National Book Awards

"Wow! A very illuminating and thought-provoking work which is both intimate and personal, yet instructive and universal. An impressive accomplishment!" —SHALENE TAKARA, editor of *Emergence of the Sensual Woman*

"Conceived in a unique act of love, Carla Tara has lived that love's unfolding in the world. Brilliant, insightful and practical, her teachings use vivid examples and practical exercises to show us how to live life authentically in love." —BRIAN BUCHBINDER, Pleasure Activist

"Those of you who have met Carla know of her courage, clarity, strength of character, and integrity. It is what makes her such an effective counselor and teacher of the mysteries of sexuality. Most importantly, she does not shy away from topics that would make some other gurus cringe. In manifesting this book, she courageously shares her life's journey, the lessons and insights, all that has made her into who she is today. She deftly weaves her personal experiences, vulnerabilities and subsequent insights into a writing that easily holds your attention, teaches, engages your intellect and most of all inspires you to see her for who she truly is. Carla is an exceptional, courageous human being, woman and tantrika." —ANTON QUON

# LESSONS FROM A

# Tantric Tango Dancer

## The High Art of Intimate Relating

## Carla Tara

Ecstatic Living Publications
New York, NY

<u>Disclaimer</u>

The information presented in this book is based on the author's personal experience. The techniques explained are to be used with the reader's discretion and ability. The author is not responsible or liable in any manner for any body sensations, experience and possible issues resulting from applying the techniques contained in this book. Success in these practices is directly related to the amount of time dedicated to them.

**Lessons from a Tantric Tango Dancer**
Copyright © 2007 by Carla Tara

Published by Ecstatic Living Publications, New York, NY

Editing by Geralyn Gendreau
Cover Photo by Daniel Cruse
Index by Betty Taylor

Daniel Cruse, Photographer
Email: AlohaPhotographer@gmail.com
Website: www.AlohaPhotographer.com

Printed in the United States of America
First Edition

ISBN 978-0-6151-4383-5

This book is dedicated to my two sons.

This Book was read for my two Sons...
This Book arrived in my life way after — I had
started my journey into the essence of being
a tandric Lover... -

This woman's heart a mind are as if —
She was me —
it was as if — I, had found my very essence
when I one day found her web-site —
I pray that I get another life — One day — to
express all that I have felt, and do feel
in my heart —

Bliss & love & life & laughter
to anyone who gets to read the Book

# Contents

*Acknowledgments*                                              iii

*Introduction*                                                  v

Chapter 1  The Forbidden Fruit                                  1

Chapter 2  The Hidden Faces of The Divine                      13

Chapter 3  The Visible Face of Eve                             27

Chapter 4  Curiosity: the Inner Teacher                        43

Chapter 5  Innocence and Imagination                           59

Chapter 6  Honesty and Sacred Communion                        81

Chapter 7  Courage and Vital Life Force                        95

Chapter 8  Trust: a Full Embrace of Life                      111

Chapter 9  Dynamic Balance                                    123

Chapter 10 Creativity and Self-Actualization                  147

Chapter 11 Make Love with the Divine                          165

*Appendices*                                                  169

# Acknowledgments

This book was inspired by Ming Fang, a passionate Argentine Tango dancer and special friend who always raises the bar and helps me reach new heights (and dips) on the dance floor.

Many important people in my life have encouraged me to write, the most influential of which is my wonderful friend Geralyn Gendreau, an award-winning editor whose keen attention helped me document the pearls that came out in our conversations. I am grateful to my friend Robert Dubiel, author of several great books, whose work as an Intuitive Psychic has guided me when my intuition was clouded by mental interference and Barnaby B. Barratt, PhD, writer and Tantra teacher, whose spiritual guidance influenced me greatly. A special thank-you goes to Maeve Fry, a great opera singer and therapist, who has been a passionate friend and counselor.

I am deeply grateful to my first Tantra teacher, Gurudev Chitrabhanu, who taught me to befriend my inner male and female, and to my many Western teachers: Lori Star, Charles Muir, Kutira DeCoster, Margo Anand, and Dr. Judy Kuriansky who has helped thousands grow into a healthier sexuality with her "Love Phones."

Deep gratitude also to my friend and star student, Vincent D'Agati, and to many dear friends who contributed to my spiritual path: Ann Gordon, Sherry Garter, Walt Sloan, Brian Buchbinder, Gary Lysak, Dr. Gary Schubach, and Thomas Casimiro. Thanks also to my Argentine Tango teachers: Paul Pellicoro, Gawain Bantle, Jim DePeyster and Dwight D. Carter who inspired me with their passion for Tango.

My deepest appreciation and thanks go to Marshal Rosenberg for his contribution to the great task of healing and reconciling human hearts with the work of Non-Violent Communication.

# Introduction

All of life is about relating. Connecting with others is a basic human need. The drive to find and feel a deep sense of belonging is quintessential to being human. Relating can be challenging, however, as early imprints from our families were not always shaped by unconditional love. Few of us have not been wounded in one way or another vis-à-vis our love nature. The impulse to heal these wounds, and to become more enlightened in our relating, compels many of us on our path of personal growth. When a sense of trust and confidence in one another flavors the relationship soup, when we know we are on the same team with another, the simple pleasure of adding to each other's joy is a delicious gift to our lives.

Our relationships with intimate partners go even further. We discuss important issues and life challenges with one another. We laugh together. We cry together. We navigate the daily chores that go into making home and hearth a warm and welcoming place to be. This is the cozy nest where we express our love and enjoy our sensual nature. If we can do this freely and enthusiastically with a sense of discovery we consider ourselves most fortunate. We gain a sense of real power from our ability to be vulnerable in another's presence. We treasure the opportunity to communicate with honesty and openness from our authentic selves. We know that nurturing the seeds of love at every turn will allow them to bloom and spread the sweet scent of that essence to all around. As we love we feel a connection that goes beyond our bodies. We start to sense that we are more than our body and become conscious of our innate connection with the divine.

Not all relationships fulfill this vision, however, and we suffer when we feel unmet or when our latent potential is not actualized. Humans form relationships and enter into marriages for all sorts of reasons. Some marry for security, some for sexual gratification, some because they feel more secure within a couple, some because they can communicate well and some because they can't and get hooked on the constant tension of trying to reach or change the other. Enlightened relationships tend to transcend all these "reasons" and have as their foundation a simple goal of growing in love and light together, whatever it takes.

During the many years I've worked as psychotherapist, relationship counselor and Tantric Healer, I have seen that any relationship—no matter how it started—can succeed as long as the partners either grow in a compatible direction or learn to tolerate and even appreciate growing in completely different directions. The key in either case is that each partner is in love with the other's essence.

Most of the couples that come to tantric therapy present some version of this complaint: we just cannot seem to fulfill each other's needs. Either the sexual expression—on the basis of which the choice to marry was made—has become stale, or the sought after safety provided by the marriage contract has become boring. One or both feel an intense, compelling longing for more sexuality and more creativity in life as well as between the sheets.

If your goal is reaching greater harmony in your relationship and a more fulfilling love life, Tantra has much to offer. A science of self-realization and a spiritual practice that enhances and transforms sexual energy to reveal its evolutionary potential, Tantra also offers practical advice for successful relationships by highlighting basic differences between man and woman or, to be more precise, between masculine and feminine energy expressions. (Throughout this book, I use the words woman and man to mean feminine expression and masculine expression; same sex partners are included and celebrated in every aspect of this discussion.)

The paradox of masculine and feminine has left many feeling as though men and women are from different parts of the galaxy altogether. Although men and women have the same basic fundamental needs for air, water, food, and affiliation with others, the masculine nature and the feminine nature are very different in their expression. Women (or the feminine in all of us) are turned on by romance; they love hearing how much they are wanted and loved. They want to hear men talk of their love and admiration for them in detail. They love romance novels and savor the more romantic passages. If men read romantic books at all (librarians say they almost never see a man picking up a romance novel) they usually skip to the juicy parts. Men are turned on by visual appearance, color of hair, the look of an outfit, the way a woman moves her head or holds her shoulders, the curve of her breast or roundness of her derriere.

Consider this example of a couple I worked with whose names—like those of all clients mentioned in this book—have been changed out of respect for privacy. When Lori came for a tantric session she complained that Don was only interested in sex. He would come home and grab her breast or her buttocks and move her toward the bedroom. Don complained that she constantly slapped his hand away, which left him feeling rejected.

"She used to like sex when we were going out," he said, exasperated.

Don was deeply confused. I asked him to remember how it was at the beginning of their relationship when Lori had been incredibly hot for him all the time. I asked him how often he had called her during the week to re-affirm his love and make plans to spend time together or arrange their next adventure. After some pondering, Don could see how his constant attentiveness had kept Lori's heart and her body open to him. He saw how his behavior allowed Lori to expand into a bigger love that translated into a greater turn

viii

on. *Feeling loved* and attended to emotionally kept her sexual urge high.

Another example of the different galaxies inhabited by the masculine and feminine can be seen in how we work through conflict. The woman (or the partner with a more feminine essence) wants to talk about what occurred until she feels truly heard. Then she can relax and open to another perspective. She can seldom be sexually open until there is a resolution. Then her heart can open and the sexual energy can flow through her body allowing for enthusiastic lovemaking. In contrast, after a fight, a man often wants to make up by making love. For the masculine, connection is more readily reestablished on a physical level rather than through talking.

Yet another stark difference is in how we experience orgasm. When a man ejaculates he emits a hormone that puts him to sleep. When women have orgasms they emit a hormone that wakes them up and increases their energy for more connection. Men who train in tantric practices learn to postpone or even withhold ejaculation. By having several subtle, energetic orgasms before ejaculating, they can stay awake and enjoy the long afterglow and pillow talk with a woman before falling asleep. This is due to the increased energy and additional charge engendered when a man transmutes the sexual spark into a blazing fire of love and devotion. That charge remains in the body even after the release of semen once a man becomes adept at this practice.

Still more differences: when women are sad, they can still be in the mood for sex, but when they are angry or tired, they are cut off from their sexual flow. Men, on the other hand, can have intercourse when they are angry and are often surprised to notice tiredness disappear when an erection emerges. While men have their highest level of testosterone in the morning, women have their highest level in the evening. (Testosterone in both sexes is largely responsible for sex drive.) Men are often ready to make love in the morning while women would rather turn over and continue to sleep.

The glorious and sexually satisfying relationship you long for requires a willingness to take our male and female differences into consideration to co-create ways to move beyond perceived limitations. A spiritually fulfilling relationship is our birthright. It takes two to Tango in the dance of life and when we move together effortlessly we evolve relationships that work. My commitment is to help you achieve an optimal way of relating based on a real understanding of yourself and another. Tantra can open you to living a state of deep connection that includes the physical and goes beyond to a state of divinity that is shared through the breath-of-life. This conscious breath of which lovers partake is the communion with the divine and the unified expression of their merging into one. Bringing this experience of Unity into daily life makes everything more alive and joyful, igniting a sacred fire that warms everyone around you.

Passion means burning with desire to live fully. Passion also means suffering through whatever bumps you come to on the road and learning to go deeper into the experience of life and therefore higher into pleasure. In Tantra we say: the deeper you go into self-knowledge the higher you can go into enlightened bliss. To get to self-knowledge requires passion. If you identify just with the light or just with the darkness, you will live a shallow life. Many of our favorite paintings are those that contain great contrasts in color. Van Gogh's work stirs the soul of anyone who has passion for life.

In the pages that follow, I will share my fascination with the myth of Eve—who I chose as my heroine at an early age. Over the years, I have drawn an analogy between the principles of a passionate life and the faces of Eve that have been hidden by the conventional, religious view of the feminine. Eve has been portrayed as the woman who disobeyed God and caused her descendants to be banished from Eden and punished by God for her original sin. From the time I was small, this idea was simply too absurd for me to swallow. By the time I was a teen, I had begun to conjure the idea that Eve had been misconstrued and that if I looked deeply I would see her real faces: curiosity, innocence, imagination, and the courage to follow your own path. Later in my life, Eve revealed ever more mature characteristics of perseverance and trust, creativity and dynamic balance.

I have come to believe that these very attributes lead to a self-actualized life—a life lived with full consciousness of both the human and divine dimensions of being. Life is a dance between the human and the divine. Perhaps this is why, in nearly every culture, people love to dance. The dance of sexual expression, emotional nakedness, and spiritual connection is the greatest joy in life. Spirit gives us the vertical dimension, and our bodies allow us to dance through life in the horizontal dimension, and the human heart center is where this union of human and divine happens.

One of my greatest teachers is Argentine Tango dancing. More than any other activity, Tango has helped me understand—and learn by doing—the give and take that allows a relationship to really work. In my work as a passionate relationship coach, this is the knowledge sought after the most. Although people come in with any number of concerns and problems, what almost every person hungers for is simple: to live in a state where conflicts and separation cease to exist and love is all there is inside and between them. Tantra acknowledges relationship as perhaps the most direct path to that goal. For only in relationship can we learn to support another, to weave between leading and following with strength, grace, and passion until we reach the point where leader and follower melt together and become the dance.

Both Tantra and Tango offer an opportunity for inner spiritual growth that affords moments of pleasure on the way to the desired enlightened state. We leave "the valley of tears" referred to in Catholic prayer behind and choose to grow through conscious presence and healthy pleasure instead of through pain. The more we grow, the closer we come to the core of who we are, and the more peace and pleasure we experience until we enter the luminous realm wherein everything disappears and only love and light shine through all of existence.

Initially, I set out to write a book about breathing. The breath is a crucial part of the healing work that I do with clients. Conscious, intentional breathing is a *resource,* one that many depleted people never realize they can tap into. Conscious breathing—with the intention to fill up with energy and spirit—is our closest ally, one that can help us recognize an enlightened state wherein we are conscious both of our divinity and our humanness, the breath being the conduit of this union.

Over time, the breathing book morphed into a discussion of the many hidden faces of Eve as mentioned above. Finally, as the story of Eve began to take shape within a larger framework, I discovered that Eve is, in essence, no different from Adam. That realization, one I had been working toward over many long years, hit me while dancing the Argentine Tango.

You need not be a Tango dancer to take up the lessons that I present in this book. The dance of life does not require music and high heels. Tantra is the art and science of weaving life into a unified whole. In Tango, that union occurs on the dance floor between man and woman. In day-to-day life, it may happen as you step off a curb on a busy street when your masculine side reaches out to lend a hand where needed at the very same moment as your feminine side is awestruck by the sheer beauty of life. Moments like these do not fail to enlighten. They humanize us and spread their vitality to every moment of our experience just as the breath does. The inhalation is the male expression, taking the breath in, and the exhalation is the feminine surrendering, absorbing the vital force and releasing what is not needed to get ready for a new breath.

Tango and Tantra will be discussed throughout these pages and utilized as both metaphor and focal point of the discussion. You need not be a dancer nor a tantrika to peel back the layers of your identity and discover the Infinite waiting to welcome you home. Adam and Eve may have been expelled from Eden in myth but Eden can be accessed once we realize it as a state of mind. Much has been said about this transition and the advances in consciousness that make it possible. Perhaps this exploration involves a reframing of our culture's central myth of the first man and woman. The "tempting" serpent could be seen as kundalini energy rising and compelling humans to become fully conscious. Adam and Eve were in a state of unconsciousness bliss, much like animals. According to the myth they did not even notice that they were naked until the snake intervened and they became conscious of duality. Eating the fruit of the forbidden tree of "good and evil" was a necessary step in our evolution. It begins the journey towards Self Realization, that comes with the *integration of the apparent opposites we know as duality.*

Bertrand Russell said, "Man is a credulous animal, he needs to believe something; in the absence of good grounds for belief, he will be satisfied with bad ones." What better use can be made of the human potential than by giving good grounding in an uplifting central myth? The hidden qualities of Eve discussed in these pages are offered as new and powerful seeds—so too, the tantric Tango lessons.

Let the dance begin.

Lessons from a Tantric Tango Dancer

# 1 The Forbidden Fruit

It has been said that well-behaved women seldom make history, and yet—for both men and women—making history is not necessarily a great prize. *Changing* history, or claiming the power to change your own life for the better, now there is a prize!

What keeps us from claiming this power is elusive. Our passion is suspect, our desires defamed. And yet we can hardly stand the feeling that constantly nudges us saying: *surely, there must be something more.*

The single act of eating an apple performed by one *misbehaving* female—the mythical Eve—has done more to shape feminine identity than perhaps any action taken by any woman since. Likewise, masculine identity is deeply influenced by the story of Adam's relationship with Eve.

Like it or not, as western men and women, we have been deeply influenced by the creation story of original sin. Yet, in the postmodern world we rarely look at our identity and emotional experience as something shaped by myth. What if I were to tell you that loneliness and depression are downstream effects directly

ated to the story of the first man and woman? What if I were to tell you that loneliness and despair are not personal? And what if I were to tell you that the antidote to loneliness and despair is equally impersonal—and readily available. Yes, readily available but not so easily recognized. Cultural conditioning predisposes us to a strange blindness where the source of happiness is concerned. We come to believe that happiness comes from outside of us, and so we "sell out". Our genuine self is sacrificed in the name of pleasing someone who will then give us the love that we have lost contact with from within. We are afraid of losing that outside love and feel guilty if we do not behave as the authorities tell us, especially if we experience passion and pleasure from it, which is forbidden. We become alienated from our true self, which is unconditional love, and habitually defend against it, unable to give or receive love without strings attached. This keeps us in a state of separation.

Separation as a state of mind and being is unnatural and contrary to our intrinsic state of enlightenment, according to Tantra. The word Tantra has its root in the Sanskrit word *tandere*, which means "to weave" and denotes interrelatedness and continuity[1]. Tantra teaches us that it is natural to be awake and in full possession of our innate love and wisdom, and that we leave that state by falling asleep—falling into toxic states of mind characterized by a lack of knowledge and awareness. These toxic states parallel the seven deadly sins—lust (Latin: luxuria), gluttony (Latin: gula), greed/avarice (Latin: cupiditia'avaritia), sloth/laziness (Latin:

---

[1] *According to the Wikipedia definition of Tantra.*

pigritia'acedia), wrath (Latin: ira), envy (Latin: invidia), and pride/hubris (Latin: superbia)—although the concept of sin is notably absent in Tantra teachings. When a person behaves in toxic ways it doesn't mean the intrinsic awakened state is not there, it simply means that he or she has lost touch with it.

To remember and fully reside in the awakened state is the aim of Tantra. The ignorance of toxic states gives way to deep self-knowledge and understanding. Our real and entirely natural need for connection and pleasure is embraced and celebrated. The student of Tantra learns to live life fully and to learn more about who we are from each experience. This learning, weaving, building, and growing process increases self-knowledge, which in turn becomes the antidote to loneliness and despair.

Both men and women are equally compelled to acquire self-knowledge. *Wanting to know* lures us toward greater understanding of self, other, and the nature of relatedness. While in search of self-knowledge, I have spent a lifetime taking two steps back but three steps forward always eventually moving toward a greater understanding of our highest potential as humans. Many of us are engaged in this search to such an extent that it becomes the driving force and the primary motivation underlying and propelling all of our activities and choices.

The hunger for knowledge is not gender specific, and in fact, invites us to find a unique inner balance of masculine and feminine when we give ourselves over to it fully. It is this inner balance that most exquisitely serves our highest potential. The first man and first woman—Adam and Eve—exist as both an *archetype* and a resource for each of us. Our newly acquired partners of wisdom and knowledge want us to be naked once again, free of fear and shame.

In many chapters of this book I relate stories from my childhood, not so much in the interest of a memoir as in the interest of evoking a certain wide-eyed innocence characteristic of a child's perspective. We had this openness in our perception before society taught us how and what to think. The intent of these stories is to trigger memories of similar experiences from your own early life. We come into this world so very *impressionable*—not at all a blank slate as once was believed but certainly moldable clay. The intent of the stories is to help you reconnect with that aspect of all of us that remains moldable despite the many glazes layered on by life experience. My intent is to engage the essential level of your being, that infinite resource we know and call forward to stimulate our growth. The stories contain feelings and images that can feed your subconscious and may well kick up memories of circumstances that you might have encountered as a child. This is their design.

We are not what society leads us to believe but rather we are much, much more. What we are is actually infinite. Whether you consult religion, philosophy, psychology, or quantum physics this is the direction in which you will be moved. Call it God, Goddess, Christ consciousness, being *saved*, the will of Allah, karma or kismet — what you have is a gorgeous invitation to expand beyond your previous limits.

*"Expanding beyond previous limits is a requirement for a healthy, vital relationship"*

Expanding beyond previous limits is a requirement for a healthy, vital relationship. As we know, relating in intimate relationships tests the self-knowledge we sometimes think we have acquired. Often reality shows we still have work to do to really embody those insights. As my beloved teacher, Gurudev Chithrabhanu used to say: "It is easy to be enlightened on a mountain top where no one bothers you. Living with someone who pushes your buttons is a different story. Your loved ones are usually *master button-pushers*; they know what triggers you. To stay awake in those moments is the true test of self-knowledge." The well-known Western guru, Ram Dass, once said that the Yoga of Relationships is the most difficult yoga of all but also the most rewarding. Key to a good relationship is to know and respect your limits and constantly check if you can go safely beyond them.

Limits are curious phenomena. Sometimes they serve our growth and sometimes they prevent it. Learning to test our limits and blast through them is just as important as learning to respect our limits. Each situation and challenge brings to bear a new moment of discovery, a moment when you can ask yourself: Is this a place where I need to back off and gather some more strength or is this a place where I need to push through? One of my favorite past-times—Argentine Tango dancing—gives me a chance to explore this edge every single week. I am often quite exhausted at the end of a day filled with sessions, exercise class, and tending to business matters. But if a Milonga—a Tango party—is happening anywhere nearby, I feel compelled to put on a favorite dress and head out for an evening of high-energy dancing. Feeling into my body, I ask, "To go or not to go?" and feel into my deeper need at the moment. Some nights I push my limits and find a second wind that carries me through an exhilarating evening. At other times, I respect my limits, take a hot bath, and surrender to my need for quiet and rest. I recognize when my body may need to heal before pushing it further.

Thus I dance between yin and yang in my own being, a good preparation for a vital relationship with another. Tango, like Tantra (the work I do as a professional yogi and passionate relationship guide), engages the masculine and feminine energies at the core of each person on a tangible level. This physical engagement yields unique insight precisely because that insight is embodied. Insight arrived at through a physical discipline is insight that can be owned. Not simply *had* in the mind and intellect but rather owned in the body. In other words, insight that changes you by expanding how you live and breathe and move about your world.

**Lesson: Understanding Limits**

Learning to evaluate your personal limits in various situations is an important part of self-knowledge and personal growth. His Holiness, the Dali Lama spoke to this in one of his speeches and the lesson he imparted never left me: we should learn the rules really well so we know which ones to follow and which ones to break.

We all have certain physical limitations that we need to consider. When we drop an object we can be certain that it will fall, even if

7

that object is our body. The law of gravity is a natural limit that affects us all in a certain clear and non-negotiable way that we all discover.

Some bodily limitations are not always quite so clear. For instance, what are your limits about staying up until the wee hours of the night? How much sleep do you need to stay healthy? How well do you know your limits in this area? How often do you choose to respect those limits? How do you feel when you go beyond your limit? I invite you to start observing the effect lack of sleep has on your body. How soon do you notice it when you're over-tired? Do you give yourself needed rest or do you tend to push through and stay up one more night?

We also have limits imposed on us by authorities: schools, government, employers, etc. See what conclusions you come to when you look back on your life with regard to this type of limit. Do you remember ever feeling like a hero when you had the courage to disregard certain outdated, useless limits that other people unconsciously follow out of fear of disobeying the authorities? Do you remember feeling good when you respected a limit that was life affirming?

Being spontaneous and creative within our limits at times can actually help us transcend those limitations and discover expanded consciousness and increased energy.

**Exercise:**

Write one example of each of the following experiences of transgressing or respecting a limit imposed on you from an outside authority:

1. You transgressed a limit and you came out feeling happy and expanded

2. You transgressed a limit and you had and unpleasant experience

3. You respected a limit and you came out feeling happy

4. You respected a limit and had an unpleasant experience

Questions to ponder:

- What where the elements that you considered to decide whether to respect or disregard a limit?

- What was the reasoning process you used to decide whether to respect that limit or not? Was the decision to disregard the limit self-serving or aimed at producing more happiness for everyone?

- Was the limit you respected one that served to provide safety for you or anyone else?

- How did you feel respecting the limit?

- How did you feel disregarding the limit?

- What made you decide to respect the limit? Was the decision a result of real thinking or did you just react?

- Did you decide to respect the limit out of fear or because you believed it was a life-serving limit?

Real thinking tested by real feelings is required to make good decisions. A good test is to ask yourself: does the choice I'm making help me feel more centered? Reactions or choices that stem from rebellion are counter-productive when the impulse is to say "no" or "yes" to what someone else is thinking rather than to think for yourself first.

"Perhaps the appeal of Tango

has much to do with what it fulfills —

our deep need for closeness and a safe haven

to move toward other people and

to relieve ourselves of isolation and separateness"

# 2 The Hidden Faces of the Divine

Walking into a Milonga, a fun Tango party, is a unique kind of high. It's no wonder that from Canada to Manhattan to Los Angeles, Tango has become quite the craze in recent years. Where else can complete strangers meet and meld their energies in total union within a social context that beautifully marries form,spontaneity and discipline with fun.Perhaps the appeal of Tango has much to do with what it fulfills — our deep need for closeness and a safe haven to move toward other people and to relieve ourselves of isolation and separateness.

The combination of discipline and pleasure is what makes Tango so compelling. Just like Tantra, Tango requires focus and dedication to the practice. Both involve a continuous stream of breath that keeps the energy between two people moving and culminates when the two become one. Few experiences are more exhilarating and potentially life changing. This type of peak

13

experience wherein two become one shows us the true potential of relationship not only as a source of great pleasure but also as a way to access the soul level where our creative genius resides.

The taboo on pleasure has been reinforced in our culture by a pervasive sex-negative mindset advanced by our major religions. For most western people, the idea that sex can be experienced and expressed as a positive evolutionary force is quite foreign. In Tantra, our most basic instinct is harnessed in just this way. The expression of sexuality as artistry comes quite naturally once the old mindset is shed. For some like me, shedding is not so difficult because we saw through the distortion from the start.

In the village where I grew up there lived two hundred people and eight hundred cows. Our little town was largely isolated from the rest of the world with only an angry river and a single road running through it leading up to a luxury ski resort high in the Italian Alps.

My brothers and I looked with envy at the rich people who passed through town on their way to a winter holiday. Few families, including ours, had enough money to buy something as frivolous as skis. Ever inventive, my brothers constructed their own simple sleds. Girls in our village were not allowed rambunctious play; our mothers insisted such things were only for boys. Never one to deny the defiant face of Eve, I broke the rule. I thought it ridiculous that only boys could tumble around in the snow. I loved the freedom of flying down a sled run on a path covered so deep with snow it came up to my eyes. Some of the boys were happy to share their sleds with me; others laughed out loud with scorn. I did not care what anybody thought; the call of freedom spoke directly to my soul.

Historically for me, Tantra grew out of this very call of freedom. In ancient times up to the present, the path of renunciation of temptation has been advanced as the primary way to realize union with God. But in Buddhism, Hinduism and Jainism, the non-renunciate tantric path grew among those who sought to find God in the simple things of day-to-day life rather than in isolated monasteries and caves. Among devout Catholics of our village simple pleasures of life were renounced altogether except for one day a year when joy and celebration were allowed. A natural tantric even then, I questioned this paradigm and aligned myself with a different path—even though decades would pass before I discovered that path had a name.

The feast day celebrating the Assumption of the Virgin Mary[2] was the single day each year that people in my village were allowed to have fun. Devotional festivities began with villagers parading through the streets holding a statue of the Madonna. All the windows throughout the village were thrown wide and draped with fine silk cloths that flapped in the warm summer breeze. People looked up at the expensive silks in awe lifting their eyes toward the sky as though it would help them see God. The family with the most valuable silks was viewed as the most pious. *How strange, I*

---

[2]*The Feast of the Assumption (Catholic): August 15th*
*It is the principal feast of the Blessed Virgin, the mother of Jesus Christ. This feast commemorates two events - the departure of Mary from this life and the assumption of her body into heaven.*
*http://www.holidays.net/dailys/holidays/assumption.htm*

thought, with mounting distrust for this odd competition. What did piety have to do with expensive silk?

The afternoon feast featured a band of horns and trumpet players; all except the very old whose hearing had gone were swept up by the gala sound. My father always stood close to the band bouncing his body up and down to the rhythm of the music, absorbed in his own private bliss.

*Why all this fuss over a woman who was a virgin?* I wondered. I had heard rumors about a priest in a nearby village falling in love with a flesh and blood woman, and I took strange comfort in his decision to put her image next to the Virgin Mary. He apparently saw the divinity in her humanness but this bold act got him dismissed from the priesthood.

Ours was a closed-minded village. People believed with great fervor that all must pay to redeem us from the sin of Eve, she who dared disobey God and become aware of good and evil. *Why would God punish awareness of anything?* I wondered. If evil as well as good exist in his Creation then shouldn't it be dealt with rather than ignored? A free thinker even then, I felt certain that Eve was a more complete woman than the Virgin Mary.

I loved the day of celebration, in spite of my confusion. My heart delighted to see my father's joy as he smiled and moved his body to the beat. My mother never showed herself among the crowd on those festive afternoons. She had enjoyed the procession and that was enough for her. Seeing this saddened me deeply and

*"Why would God punish awareness of anything?"*

at eight years old I decided never to become as serious-minded as my mother. I wanted to be like my father and freely express my joy. *Life should be a celebration,* I thought. That people waited to celebrate life only a few days a year seemed absurd.

In this look at the various faces of Eve I include her consort, Adam, in the discussion.

The qualities we will look into are not gender-specific and can be cultivated by both women and men. Likewise, both women and men are engaged in the development of higher conscious awareness that I believe to be the deeper meaning behind Eve's act of eating the forbidden fruit. While looking at the story of Adam and Eve from a perspective of higher consciousness we will take into account the masculine and feminine energies that exist within each individual regardless of gender. For example, we could say that picking the fruit from the Tree of Knowledge was an act performed by Eve's masculine *provider* aspect. The inner decision to do so was made by her feminine aspect. To her consciousness as a whole, enraging the "authority" was worth the risk involved.

Growing up in a small village taught me to have strong inner will. Just like Eve, I chose my own destiny rather than comply with the expectations of the "authority." There is a difference between inner and outer willpower. Outer willpower has external goals: to achieve, to compete, to climb the ladder. Inner willpower arises naturally out of self-knowledge and is always aligned with our soul purpose. Inner willpower, once developed, can merge with the softness of the heart and give birth to creative intelligence. This powerful combination transforms an ordinary human into

In the minds of those interested in maintaining the sta

creators can be perceived as a threat. And yet our deeper nature wants to be expressed and will rise in certain individuals regardless of suppressive forces. The natural Tantrics and Tantrikas of the world, are those who like Eve, cannot help but oppose anything that seems to be life stifling and repressive to their nature.

Eve's apparent face—that of the disobedient woman who disregards God's command—is called into question here. According to the story, the serpent tempted Eve to disobey. This interpretation forms the cornerstone of a conventional, puritanical worldview in which the duality of "good and evil" is accepted as gospel. The Catholic Church has used this interpretation to gain followers; according to their dogma, being baptized is the only way to erase Eve's "original sin" and open the road to salvation. Consider for a moment a wholly different referential system. In yoga, the snake is a symbol for Kundalini, the evolutionary force that lies coiled at the base of the spine in the area of the perineum. This force needs to be awakened to reach enlightenment. Viewed through this frame of reference, we can understand that the snake is not so much tempting Eve (and us) into evil as it is nagging us to reach for and actualize the evolutionary potential of consciousness we are all born with. When kundalini starts to awaken through self-knowledge, it moves up the spine activating higher functions in energy centers known as the *chakras*. As

*"When kundalini starts to awaken through self-knowledge, it moves up the spine activating higher functions in energy centers known as the chakras."*

kundalini journeys from chakra to chakra, we gain access to better health, more balanced personal power, greater connection, deeper love, higher intelligence, and finally the fullness of our innate divinity.

The chakras are vortexes of energy that move like wheels, absorbing and distributing energy throughout the body to keep us healthy and vibrant. The chakras also store extra energy in order to supply the body's needs in periods of stress. Men often fall asleep after ejaculation if they have not learned to store energy in their chakras during lovemaking. In this case when men *come* they actually *leave!*

In my re-interpretation of the creation story, Eve was not defying or trying to outsmart God. She was looking to discover her own innate divinity. But she knew that her real face must be kept hidden until the time is right. The journey to become conscious of one's deeper nature is a secret one. Once fulfilled, the Eve in each woman can proudly express her many hidden faces to the world. Like a diamond that shines its beauty through many facets, each of Eve's hidden faces reflects the inner divine core. Together, these many faces form the brilliant diamond that she has worked to embody.

The brilliant faces of Eve that shine through her passion for truth and awareness are:

curiosity
- innocence with imagination
- courage
- creativity
- honesty
- trust
- and balance

One of the primary legacies of the myth of Adam and Eve is the experience of shame. When the first man and woman *sinned* their nakedness was exposed and the essential self—that innocent, courageous, creative radiance at the core of each being—went into hiding. The repression of sexual energy led to many taboos against expressing erotic love. Our basic nature became twisted out of shape. Few cultures have successfully managed the sexual force. In ancient India, sexuality was far more integral to society. This is not to say that the sexual force was fully integrated and harnessed for the good but more varied attempts were being made.

Tantra is becoming more and more known in the West and is both a science and an art that guides us to use all of our energies, including our sexual energy to live a more intimate, expanded, and fulfilling life on our way to enlightenment. These energies are woven first within our bodies, then back and forth to and from the body of a lover, going higher and higher in an ecstatic spiral of multiple orgasms leading to the highest Orgasm of all—the merging in love with God/Goddess. The German word for Orgasm, *die Klimax*, means Stairway to Heaven.

*"Tantra is becoming more and more known in the West*
*and is both a science and an art*
*that guides us to use all of our energies, including our sexual*
*energy to live a more intimate, expanded, and fulfilling life*
*on our way to enlightenment"*

Some tantric masters have successfully utilized Tantra to reach Enlightenment, that ultimate union we all long to achieve. Union is the deepest consummation of love. As Pierre Teilhard de Chardin said so beautifully, "The day will come after harnessing the ether, the winds, the tides, gravitation, we shall harness for God the energies of love. And, on that day, for the second time in the history of the world man will have discovered fire."

## Lesson: Becoming Aware of Shame

In Tantra classes, I often take participants through the following exercise to help reveal the fallacy of shame. Many of us who were raised with a sex-negative mindset have had our self-concept colored by shame. A potent distortion of the essential self, culturally induced shame limits our self-expression. This simple exercise is designed to help you see through the distortion of shame and simply be aware of your humanness. This exercise is best done with a partner but if a partner is not available then simply engage your active imagination and bring the presence of another to mind.

- Sit face to face with a partner.
- Call to mind your deepest, darkest secret.
- Imagine revealing this secret to the person sitting across from you. Notice the feelings that come up for you.
- Notice the stories you tell yourself about what this person will think of you once they know your secret. How do you imagine that they will see you and feel about you once they know your secret?

- Now imagine that you are hearing the person across from you tell you exactly the same secret about him or her self.
- Notice if your feelings for this person change. Do your feelings about them change significantly?
- Decide whether or not to reveal your secret. Whatever you decide will be perfect.

A very high percentage of my students who did this exercise in a workshop setting were surprised to find that they felt more trust in the person after they revealed their secret than they had before. Furthermore, after revealing their own "dark" secret they actually felt relieved of the burden they did not for the most part realize they'd been carrying.

**Exercise:**

- Remember what your parents and parent substitutes, your first *gurus*, taught you about sex either implicitly or explicitly. Write it down.
- What did you learn about sex from other "teachers" including boys and girls your age?
- How was your fist sensual experience when you first touched yourself?
- How was your first sexual experience with another person?

Write as much as you can remember.

If what you learned from your parents or parent substitutes and/or if your first sexual experiences where negative you likely had some shame mixed into your growing sense of yourself as a sexual being. Several of my clients started to reclaim the fullness of their sexuality following these steps: (you may find that different steps might work better for you.)

- admitting to yourself the negative programming you were not completely aware of before
- writing down this programming in as much detail as possible
- getting all the cells of your bodies engaged in the healing by breathing the Ocean Breath[3] to stir up the pot,
- feel all the feelings and
- achieve complete relaxation by opening to an unconditional love connection with yourself.

---

[3] *See Lesson: Ocean Breath pg. 55*

# 3   The Visible Face of Eve

Not until I reached the age of forty did I glimpse the profound effect of what occurred the night my parents conceived me. Little had changed in our small village during the many years I'd lived abroad. My family and the villagers seemed somehow suspended in the eighteenth century. I was on a mission to understand my roots and fate played its hand when a nasty fall on an icy stairway left me with a broken leg. Forced to keep my leg immobilized for ten days, a rare opportunity emerged. Since it was deep into winter, my mother was not absorbed in the daily farm chores that would have kept her busy in warmer months. As we sat across a big wooden table in the kitchen drinking tea, my mother and I began to talk.

Being a psychotherapist with good listening skills and a solid understanding of the human psyche, I knew our conversations would be enhanced if my mother felt safe to reveal herself. With considerable effort, I managed to stay silent and not answer back when she made comments that would have triggered a major reaction in me in the past. I wanted to find out as much as I could about my background so I held my tongue and gently probed. After several days of this, we came around to the most difficult conversation of all and began to talk about sex.

"Mother, why do you suppose I am so different from my brothers and sisters?"

She sighed and reflected thoughtfully. After a few long moments, she began to speak softly, all the while looking down and not at me. "It must be because of what happened the night that I became pregnant with you. Your father had just come home from the convent where he'd been invited to taste the wines. It was like he was like a different man. He looked at me with a look I'd never seen before. It was as if he really saw me for the first time. I liked the way he touched me that night. He was very relaxed which allowed me to feel more relaxed as well. I imagine it was also the wine; your father was not accustomed to drinking. We started making love I felt pleasure with sex for the first and only time in my life. I felt the morning nausea very soon after that. I knew that I had become pregnant that night because we did not make love after that for a long time."

I was stunned to think that my mother had only enjoyed sex on one occasion in her entire life but kept this to myself and gave her a chance to speak. She continued, "When I became pregnant with your brothers and sisters I did not feel pleasure. Sex is something a

28

woman is supposed to do; having pleasure during sex is a sin. I was afraid for you because of it, afraid that my sin allowed the devil to enter into the child. When I got confirmation that I was pregnant, I prayed that I would be able to abort. I all but stopped eating but God did not listen to my prayers. You were born the following spring."

I swallowed a couple of times as I integrated this news. She looked at me expectantly waiting for comment.

"It must have been very difficult for you to have that fear your entire pregnancy."

She nodded, obviously relieved.

Encouraged by her honesty and willingness to talk about this forbidden subject, I sensed the time was right to bring up another. "Mother, do you remember that day I came down from the pasture quite upset and crying?" That day was one neither of us would ever forget for it changed the shape of our family forever. I was thirteen at the time and shortly thereafter ran away from home.

I sat there with my leg propped up on a chair and watched my mother's face contract. As I'd hoped, she felt safe enough to allow the memories to come. Her eyes opened wide as she dropped her mouth in exactly the face I saw all those years ago when I first stumbled into the kitchen and told her my brother had pushed me to the ground and forced himself inside me. But this time, she spoke, "Oh, my God, I am so sorry! Please forgive me, Carla."

I never imagined hearing those words from my mother. Tears were in both our eyes as we hugged.

She did not explain much except to say, "I was afraid of your brother. He looked and behaved so much like my father whom I always feared greatly."

She said little else. My deepest fear—that she thought that I was to blame—suddenly lost its power. The question of *fault* no longer mattered. What had happened simply happened. At that moment the visible face of Eve—the one who is to blame and must forever hide behind her shame—disappeared from mind and my world. And more importantly, I felt closer to my mother than ever in my life. A warm feeling that I had never felt before in her presence permeated my body.

My mother, like so many of her generation, had completely absorbed the prevailing Roman Catholic belief that pleasure during sex is a sin. She never questioned this belief and internalized a negative image of God. For her, God demanded work and sacrifice; pleasure was for the hereafter. The God of her imagining loved martyrs. God was precisely like her father in many ways. She had no warmth from or for her father and could feel no warmth for or from God, only fear.

When I was a girl, my mother would occasionally start to sing and fill the evening air with old-country ballads. My younger sister and I would join in the chorus. My mother looked beautiful when she sang and her joy filled the room with golden light. But after an hour or so, she would abruptly stop. As if caught doing something bad, she would say, "Oh my God, what will happen tomorrow because we had such a good time today?" This anti-pleasure

*"The God of her imagining loved martyrs.*
*God was precisely like her father in many ways"*

position colored every aspect of my mother's life and as such became a self-fulfilling prophecy.

When she came to visit me in New York, I took great pleasure in showing my mother around the city. We went to Broadway shows and fine restaurants. She enjoyed all kinds of food that she had never tasted before. When I took her to an amusement park she behaved like a little girl and even mounted a little horse on the carousel. Every once in a while, the visible face of Eve would come forward and she would say, "Oh, my God! Something bad is going to happen. I am having too much fun here."

When she went back to Italy three weeks later Mother found her bedroom completely flooded. A water pipe on the top floor had broken and nobody noticed until it was too late. All her important papers and mementos had been destroyed. Even the bed and linens had to be thrown away. This was—in her mind—God's punishment: she was a bad girl for having had too much fun.

Little did my mother know that when she exclaimed, "Oh, my God, something bad is going to happen!" she had uttered one of most powerful prayers of all. So certain that she deserved punishment, the kinetic energy of her mind attracted the circumstance almost instantaneously. Curious to know if my theory was true, I asked her to find out precisely when the water pipe broke. Sure enough, it broke on the very day she spoke her *prayer.*

My mother spent so much time on her knees reciting the conventional "Hail Mary," and "Our Father," that she grew large callous-like growths that had to be surgically removed. But pray as

32

she might, the time spent on her knees never brought the immediate results of her emotional prayer that day. Why? On an emotional level she did not believe she deserved God's ear; emotionally she *knew* that she was a sinner. Every prayer was marbled with doubt. Her fear—or better yet, her certainty—that God would not help a sinner like her sabotaged every single prayer.

This incident with the water pipes made such a strong impression on me that I began paying closer attention to my own unconscious prayers. Whenever I catch myself sending out some version of the pipe-breaking command then I immediately cancel the negative prayer.

Paying attention to what we tell ourselves is vital. Repeated thoughts become affirmations. When strong emotion accompanies repetitive thoughts then they can become powerful prayers.

Mark and Liza, a couple that I treated in therapy, come to mind as an example of the power of unintentional prayers. Fearing she had lost her libido and could no longer be a good lover to her husband, Liza repeatedly told herself, "I cannot feel anything!" Exasperated by the sudden shift in their sex life, Mark began to wonder if her complaint about not being able to feel was just a smokescreen. In an individual session he told me, "I'm starting to think she has another lover and this is just a story to cover that up."

In her solo session Liza assured me she did not have another lover. "Why would I take a lover? Having a husband is hard enough when I've lost the ability to feel. Every time he touches me I feel pressured to respond the way I used to. I feel like a total failure as a woman!" Liza's fear had turned into a negative prayer.

During therapy we discovered that Liza had absorbed her mother's strong belief that sex becomes a low priority after people get married. On countless occasions her mother's belief had been clearly spelled out: "Your husband will calm down after getting married. You will stop feeling sexy after a couple of years. By that time you will have bound your husband to you with a child. Once you have his child he's not going to divorce you because it would cost him too much money. You then can put all your attention to your child and raise it the way you want."

Liza did not have a child yet but she'd been married for two years and was hoping to become pregnant soon. She continued having sex although her feelings were gone. The focus of sex was on having a child; no longer was sex a source of pleasure. Liza hid this from her husband and kept her feelings and her mother's teaching her secret.

The message from her mother was a dangerous one and yet Liza had ingested it completely. Her mother's belief had become her unconscious prayer. Once she could see this we worked out a way to demagnetize that *prayer* and she started to regain access to her feelings.

Sexual dysfunctions such as Liza's are quite common.

Those affected by them often hide their problem out of shame and this, unfortunately, compounds the problem. Sexual dysfunctions are more common than most of us realize. Thinking "there is something wrong with me" we hide the problem. In contrast, few of us would feel ashamed or tend to hide a problem with our heart or our liver. We might be sad or fearful, but feelings of embarrassment and shame would not prevent us from seeking professional help.

The most common sexual dysfunctions in men are: loss of desire, erectile dysfunctions, premature ejaculation and impotence. Women are more likely to experience inhibited sexual desire, lack of orgasm, insufficient lubrication and painful intercourse. According to the Journal of the American Medical Association in 1999 more than 100 million Americans reported struggling with chronic sexual dysfunctions and many of them were not aware that there is help available. (see Appendix G for more information and resources). A single lesson in breath awareness and circular breathing can be a powerful tool to resolve most problems related to lack of energy and anxiety during lovemaking. Habitual shallow breathing fills only the upper part of the chest where the lungs are narrow and smaller. The bottom of the lungs is far more richly supplied with large veins and therefore more oxygen can be transferred to the blood.

To be fully present energetic lovers, we need to breathe deeply to facilitate this exchange as fully as possible. Tantra teaches different breaths for different purposes. Breath awareness is crucial for extended lovemaking that leads to higher states of conscious awareness. Many sexual dysfunctions are related to emotional issues and Tantra addresses these as well. Often, entrenched negative communication habits, unspoken resentments, and old hurts build a

*"Breath awareness is crucial for extended lovemaking*

*that leads to*

*higher states of conscious awareness"*

cold wall between lovers. Unconscious issues can come screaming to the surface in love relationships. A good Tantric Healer can help you look at these issues and give you powerful tools to release blocks and resolve unfinished issues that limit the joy of lovemaking.

When our issues are repressed and feelings are rationalized rather than felt, the unexpressed emotions form blocks along the pathways where orgasmic energy would otherwise flow throughout the body. Men especially suffer from societal conditioning that compels them to repress or rationalize feelings rather than experience their emotions. When such blocks are active, a man's vitality is lower and sex becomes more a "squeeze and burst" event, a letting go of tension rather than an intimate sharing of love and pleasure enjoyed for the sake of deepening the bond and with another.

In a world where sex is polarized as either shameful by religionists or shameless by pornographers, some men have developed a technique repertoire designed to "make her come" with the goal of being able to ejaculate without feeling—or being viewed as—selfish, or inattentive. Unfortunately, this shortsighted solution leaves the opportunity for emotional connection and deeply fulfilling lovemaking lost somewhere between the sheets. The immediate relief robs both partners of the opportunity to enjoy lovemaking as an experience of deep heart connection and nurturing. Lovers thus deprive themselves of deeper and longer pleasure that enlivens all the cells of the body.

In a tantric context, making love is a celebration that literally *makes love* grow in the interest of living a longer, happier life on the way to enlightenment. Tantra proposes using the powerful fuel of sexual energy to reach enlightenment rather than suppress it and reach for the divine through renunciation.

Mystics of many religions, in their attempts to describe the state of enlightenment, have used terms that just as readily describe a tantric orgasm such as: merging in complete union with all of life, a liberating plunge into the eternal NOW, ending the illusion of a linear continuity between past and future created by the ego in order to maintain its identity, complete freedom from concerns about survival, being infused with joyful lightness and a powerful peace that "passes all understanding."

For most of us, orgasm is a great release from ego entanglements and projection; for those short moments in time we are free of the mind's interference. No one thinks about what they should do or should have done during an orgasm. In a tantric orgasm we 'hang out' with God –that is, all of life as One—much longer than during a regular orgasm. Tantra elevates sexual experience to a level of transcendence. The ego ceases to exist, and in its place a peaceful, blissful merging with everything occurs where sound and light become one single expression of this Union. That is how you can feel when you know how to transmute sexual energy into its highest potential.

Breath is one of the main four keys that unlock this potential in Tantra. The other three are sound, movement and meditative intention.

Deep breathing helps bring emotions to the surface. "E-motion" is derived from the Latin *exmovère*, which literally means moving out. Emotions are energies in motion. When emotions are felt, sexual energy can reach higher levels riding higher and wider waves sending into ecstatic lovemaking that is really fulfilling. Sex without emotions leaves people tired, empty and sometimes even sad. We instinctively know there is much more that we can experience from an orgasm.

Deep breathing is also a key to avoiding anxiety about performance. When your whole body tingles with aliveness and you hear your lover breathe equally deeply, perhaps even making a sound on each exhalation, you are less prone to thinking about performance and more about riding the waves of pleasure a little longer.

Tantra offers the view that we are *spiritual beings* having a physical experience and thus have infinite potential for expressing love. By adding a spiritual dimension to the lovemaking, we elevate mere sex to a place where sexual ecstasy opens the door to infinite creativity. As spiritual beings we have unlimited potential and boredom is no longer a danger.

In the following chapters we are going to discover the faces of Eve that she had to hide in shame. They are: curiosity, innocence, courage, creativity, honesty, trust and balance.

Passion and compassion are the basis on which the whole process of rediscovery and ownership of those qualities is based. Compassion is actually the embodiment of divine love that Tantra moves us toward. In fulfilling my lover's needs an energy exchange takes place and my own needs are fulfilled as well.

### Lesson: Unearthing the Sex-Negative Mindset

Unearthing our sex-negative mindset is of utmost importance. Only after discovering the negative believes we might have absorbed do we have the power to choose to change them.

### Exercise:

- Buy or rent the movie *Kama Sutra*. As you watch the film, take note of the differences between a culture that embraces sexuality rather than represses it.
- Then search for your own prevalent attitudes about sexuality.
- Write down the beliefs you absorbed growing up.
- Notice how you talk to yourself about your sexual desire and feelings.
- Write down some of your favorite ways to restrict yourself
- Become aware of what you've learned about sex from your family
- Make a list of what you have learned about sex in general
- Consider each belief that you have absorbed. Is this still your belief? If you say NO very fast you may only be

looking at your surface thoughts. Consider if
might have changed your intellectual understanc
have some deep-seated beliefs to uncover.

- Is it possible that in certain highly energetic mo. ...ts the emotional component of those beliefs will still show up to interfere with your highest potential for pleasure?

- To make sure you really have updated your beliefs about sex look at your life. Your reality will give you feedback as to whether you still have negative or restrictive beliefs hiding beneath conscious awareness.

- Buy or rent a copy of *The Secret*. This DVD graphically depicts how The Law of Attraction works in our lives. This enjoyable and well- documented program could easily be part of a "How Life Really Works" course.

- Remind yourself that it takes time to attract the new reality into your life that is consistent with your new beliefs and revised thoughts. So be patient and consistently aware of small changes in the new direction.

- Periodically take stock of what's so and encourage yourself to continue on the path to full consciousness and freedom.

Start a journal and write down what you observe see on your inner map of reality; you will become more and more aware the more time you spend in self-observation. Some negative beliefs remain hidden behind the conscious thoughts that are usually more current and more liberal. This journal is the place where you will author your own central myth.

# 4   Curiosity: The Inner Teacher

To my child's eyes, my mother was the most beautiful woman in the world. When she said that I was ugly I believed her. Perhaps I *was* the devil's child as she feared. My straight hair and high cheekbones were nothing like those of my sister whose round face and curly hair were so perfect in my mother's eyes. My eyes were so large they looked almost freakish. Was I somehow allied with the dark side? Perhaps that explained why I asked so many questions my mother did not know how to answer.

Mother was more interested in work than knowledge. To her way of thinking most of my questions were *stupid* because they did not refer to work or to things she could observe. This work ethic clouded her maternal instinct and even overrode it at times. Only a mother with a one-track mind would dismiss a sick child after a quick glance and brush of her forehead saying, "No blood, no fever, go to work."

My mother wore the visible fallen face of Eve: the sinful woman whose only job is repentance through work, work, work, and more work. Rest for my mother was equivalent to laziness and laziness, according to her father, was at the root of all vices. But my passion for knowing burned inside me and my father fed that passion with his gentle and also curious nature. *His* religion made perfect sense to me.

I might ask my mother, "Why do you go to church every morning even when there is ice on the road and you could hurt yourself? If God is omnipresent then can't he hear your prayers anywhere?"

And she would simply say, "Stop asking stupid questions."

My father's religion, on the other hand, had common sense answers that were straightforward and clear.

"Why do you not go to church like mamma?" I asked him in the pasture one day.

"Because I think that God is more like the sun than a human being. When the sun is out, I am happy. I think God wants us to be happy."

That made more sense to me than the entire catechism.

My father's religion was simple and grounded in the natural world. From him, I learned the deeper laws of nature and the power of love. He taught me that singing to the cows caused them to give more milk long before science proved it to be a fact. He taught me through example that animals feel your love for them and will actually respond to your call.

I put this into practice to see if it were true. I loved each cow and would call each one by name as I gently caressed her neck. When I stretched out my open hand, the cows loved to lick up the saltiness of my skin. This is how I bonded with the cows and eventually learned to pasture ten at once without a stick. If the cows began to stray from the field then I would simply call their names and watch them come back.

The power of love was one of my first *big discoveries*. And the experience of that firsthand knowing increased my thirst for learning. Tantra directs us to seek direct knowledge through experience. Intellectual understanding acquired from books or lectures can give us a quick mental boost but fails to deliver whole-body wisdom the way a juicy experience of reality can. Real knowledge comes when we follow our natural curiosity and explore on a physical level the ideas we have grasped with our intellect.

My great desire for knowledge did not meet its match until I reached the fourth grade. Giuliana was an unusually gifted elementary school teacher. In her classroom, my questions were met with great enthusiasm. Unlike my mother, this woman thought my questions were brilliant and they clearly stimulated her excitement and desire to impart knowledge to me.

So deep was my love for this teacher that my heart would leap when I looked at her. I still remember her fragrance. I did not know it then but she was my first love—a love that was passionate and relaxing at the same time. This love was for knowledge and for the women who embodied knowledge. Hers was the first hidden face of Eve to reveal itself to me: curiosity. The knower and what became known through her merged into a passionate, but in no way sexual, love. I did not know what was happening but a tingling sensation filled my body every time she answered my questions. I wanted to be like her. This curious side of Eve was the essence I longed for but found no trace of in my own mother.

When my teacher read us a story or a poem she spoke in a wonderful voice that conveyed emotion. Love, courage, joy, and sadness, all were stirred up when she read these stories. I often awoke at four o'clock in the morning to study the poems and learn to recite them with similar emphasis. When Giuliana read fine literature such as *I Promessi Sposi* by Manzoni, my eyes would widen and become moist. I was touched both by the story's content and by her delivery. I could not wait to go to school in the morning. I felt happy and relaxed in school, a state of being I never felt in my family.

I wanted to grow up and be like my teacher, to be able to help people feel the sensations I felt and increase their knowledge at the same time. What a gift! Perhaps God was more like Giuliana than the God in Heaven described by the priest in Catechism class. Perhaps God was really a Goddess as well.

"Every human being senses an inner longing that goes deeper than the longings for emotional and creative fulfillment. This longing comes from sensing that another more fulfilling state of consciousness and a larger capacity to experience life must exist." (Pathwork Guide Lecture 204)

When it rained on the farm we could not go out to work in the fields so I would look for a place to hide from my mother and sister where I could be alone to think and dream.

One day, I finally got my courage up and climbed to the attic. It seemed a perfect place to be with my vivid imagination undisturbed. I crawled up on a dangerously shaky wooden ladder, holding my breath so as not to feel the fear. When I finally reached the top, I slowly slid open the old door. A very loud scream—that scared even me—came out of my throat. I lost my balance and nearly fell off the top of the ladder as a flurry of mice scattered away. I was not afraid of cows but mice stirred up revulsion in me. However, the revulsion I felt was immediately erased by what hit my nose. To this day I can smell it, the powerful odor of *old*. How long had that pile of books been hidden away in the attic out of reach to all but a family of mice?

Curiosity once again took over and dispelled all my fears. What secrets might be contained in those books? I remembered some vague family story about a crazy great uncle who collected books. Might they contain the answers I was searching for? Might they solve the mystery of: *Who is God? Why are we born? How do people beyond my village think?*

Trembling, I picked up the book on top and read the title: *La Gerusalemme Liberata* (The Freed Jerusalem). It smelled musty but that did not bother me. Unlike the books we read in school, this one was written in verses. Immediately, the story drew me in; it was the story of the Crusades. Many words I'd never seen before and I had to guess at their meaning. Reading quickly, I skipped through the parts about the Holy War; the idea that war could be holy made no sense to_me. What drew me in were the descriptions of how the men felt as they discovered new ways of thinking while living in exotic lands. Many of the stories told of the great passion felt by the crusaders for exotic women they met on their travels. I began to dream of an armored knight loving me the way the crusaders loved and adored these ladies who were typically unattainable women. In my innocence, I conjured the notion that a knight would love me even more because I could be had. Little did I know that their passion was stirred by the very fact that the woman was out of reach and often already married.

Thus, at a young age, I had my first encounter with the Madonna-Whore split. The unattainable woman was definitely the Madonna. Where was the real woman, the one who loved sex? Why was she considered less important than the woman who hovered above it all? Of course, I did not recognize this at the time; pattern recognition came much later. As a child I simply thought it strange and this fed my curiosity even more.

For the better part of a month I spent every moment I could steal from the farm chores and my mother's watchful eye reading that book. When I was finished I climbed back to the attic and once again scanned the mysterious stack of books. One particular book seemed to almost pull my hand toward it: *The Divine Comedy* by

Dante Alighieri. I loved the title and imagined that I would fir
discover God's sense of humor. *Now here is a book that might answer my
questions!* I thought.

Little did I know the book was a classic—more a philosophical
cosmology than an actual comedy. As the first book written in the
Latin dialect spoken in Italy, its publication elevated Italian to a pure
language.

I devoured the book and the prevailing paradigm. Fascinated by
Dante's vivid description of hell, purgatory and paradise, two
distinct revelations occurred for me while reading that book. The
first was Dante's depiction of a number of popes in hell, which
deeply satisfied my sense of justice and confirmed my suspicion that
popes were not infallible.

Even more important to my subsequent development is that, in
the end, Dante comes face-to-face with God Himself and is granted
understanding of Human nature. That such understanding was
possible for Dante set up an expectation in me at a very early age
that I would eventually have the boon as well.

Understanding comes through unexpected doors and in unlikely
forms. One of the most surprising *teachers* I've come across is the
practice of Argentine Tango. In fact, my fascination with Eve
reached its culmination in "The Tantra of Tango." A unique yoga in
its own right, Tango is as complete a system for understanding
human connection as any I have come across. The beauty—and
perhaps a good deal of the power of Argentine Tango—lies in the
simple fact that self-expression and fun are the goals. A structured

dance from that allows infinite creativity where partners connect heart to heart with great passion.

Tango invites a unique form of Tantra.

Throughout the Argentine Tango dance there is a relaxed focus on the heart connection. Just as in Tantra when lovers merge into one, in Tango, the dancers become one heart-to-heart. When the two enter into the ecstasy of the dance they are no longer doing steps but becoming the dance and the light of each other's essence becomes visible. Those watching are often left breathless and in awe.

Paradoxically, the intensity of our focus on a certain goal can keep it out of reach. If you've ever looked into the night sky to find the Pleiades you know what I mean. Looking directly at the constellation all but ensures the stars cannot be seen. However, when you look at the space around them with an off-point gaze then the constellation appears.

Likewise, by focusing intently on the dance, Tango offers a rare and beautiful opportunity to experience full union with another. The partners may not even know each other but the dance affords a structure in which to experience a passionate connection with another human being. Stirred by the music and the closeness of the heart, the emotional energy of the dance builds to lift the partners up and out of their ordinary state.

Any art form has the potential to carry us higher into a state wherein we experience our innate union with all that is. Curiosity, as your inner teacher, can lead you to precisely those forms of dance

*"Throughout the Argentine Tango dance*
*there is a relaxed focus on the heart connection.*
*Just as in Tantra when lovers merge into one, in Tango,*
*the dancers become one heart-to-heart"*

or other self expression that will unlock your hidden potential. Crucial to the process of actualizing that potential is increasing your capacity to simply be aware, and the most immediate means to that end is literally as close as your next breath.

Focused, deliberate breathing unites our emotional, sexual, and spiritual energy. Breathing is life. We can live for forty days without food, five days without water, but only a few minutes without air. Quick, shallow breathing increases alertness in the short run but leads to over-excitement and anxiety in the long run. Slow, deep breathing evokes a sense of calm and a detached viewpoint, a state of mind and being that allows us to immediately get in touch with our power and love, a place from which we can act both courageously in the face of obstacles and more deeply loving with another.

Unlike many breath control exercises, deep belly breathing is not controlled at all. Belly breathing is actually a misnomer, but I like to use this term because it reminds us to allow our belly to move down toward the sexual center. A more precise but less poetic term for this practice would be deep diaphragmatic breathing. With this type of full, relaxed inhalation the diaphragm pushes the belly out of the way for the lungs to fill up fully at the bottom where most of the venous blood is located, thus increasing oxygenation. This is the natural breath that babies breathe; we all breathe this way when we fall asleep. Stress, socialization, and a variety of other pressures push our breath into the upper part of our lungs.

The mind body split that values thinking and reason over feeling and emotion is reinforced each time we take a shallow, cut-off breath. Slow, deep breathing allows us to return to our wholeness to see with our intuition as well as our rational mind. From this place we can connect with a partner in a more balanced and compassionate way and prepare our bodies for the highest spiritual ecstasy.

Breath awareness and full belly breathing also helps heighten sexual awareness and pleasure. Too often we approach sex with a goal orientation where reaching orgasm is the aim. This leads to dissatisfaction when the goal is reached too soon or not at all. Breathing for sexual arousal and connection expands the pleasure of lovemaking far beyond the simple act of intercourse. Deep belly breathing opens the channels for full body orgasms. The euphoric state of deep lovemaking can be sustained for hours rather than minutes with simple breath awareness.

Open-mouth breathing especially slows down the mind. The more relaxed you are in the jaw and throat, the more your sex center and your nervous system can relax. This opens a direct connection between the heart and the head and allows your attention to move into the lower body. Pleasure increases as sensation increases. The rational mind gives less interference in the form of judgment and comparison when we practice full belly breathing. Your natural curiosity will come forward when you let go of what you know and step into the infinite possibilities of each new moment.

### Lesson: Peak Experience

The most important tools nature has given us to reach peak experiences are:

- the use of your breath in a conscious way,
- the ability to focus your mind on the moment,
- the ability to open your heart
- the ability to be spontaneous and creative
- making sounds and
- moving the body fluidly

### Exercise:

- I'm inviting you to reflect on a time when you had some kind of *peak experience* that carried you beyond your known self.
- Trace what led you to that moment.
- See if you can find the thread of curiosity and spontaneity that led you there.

## Lesson: Tantric Ocean Breath[4]

This is the feminine, Shakti breath, not a controlled breath like many yogic pranayamas that focus mainly on nose breathing, counting the seconds we take to inhale and exhale, and sometimes holding the breath in or out the lungs a certain number of seconds. These controlled yogic breaths are masculine in nature. They are mainly used to direct the energy from the lower chakras—the sex and power centers—to the upper chakras, which correspond to the heart, throat, third eye, and crown. This intentional raising of the energy transforms the vital force so that it can fuel higher love and carry us into a state of divine union. The cobra breath is one such masculine or Shiva breath; in a tantric context, a man can use this practice to completely transform his sexuality. Men who master this form of focused breathing can experience whole body orgasms without ejaculation. When such an orgasm is achieved the orgasmic energy spreads to all the cells of the body and moves the lovers into a state of ecstatic union.

The Ocean Breath is best taken with open mouth. When the mouth is open the breath can more readily fill and expand the bottom of the lungs and thus fill you up with more energy while you are remaining relaxed, a state that allows for deep connection both with your own feelings and the feelings of your lover. Connection is much easier with mouth open; you are always a step closer to kiss and it's easier to make sounds.

---

[4] *See also Appendix D*

<u>Try it for yourself:</u>

- Take 10 breaths with your nose while looking into the mirror.
- Then take 10 breaths gently opening your mouth
- Notice your facial expression during the first and the second practice.
- Is your face more open and relaxed when you are breathing with your nose or with your mouth?
- Is your energy higher when you do nose breathing or mouth breathing?

**Exercise:**

- Lie down comfortably on the floor on your back with your knees bent and your feet flat on the floor. Watch your breathing for several moments. Notice if you tend to breathe with your upper chest or with your diaphragm.
- Start the practice by allowing your mouth and jaw to relax open as you breathe in and out. Use active visualization and imagine your body as the ocean. Watch the waves of your breath go up and down like swells on the sea. Your inhalation is the wave rising, and your exhalation is the wave falling back once more into the ocean.
- Put your hands on your abdomen and begin to breathe, allowing your abdomen to expand naturally as the wave comes up without forcing it. Feel your hands rise up with the wave as you inhale and fall as the wave recedes into the

ocean on your exhale, allowing your belly to fall toward your back. Just intend the air to fill your belly up and let your trunk expand as much as it wants

- Take deep breaths and gently allow your belly to rise with inhalation and fall with exhalation. Make sure you don't control the exhalation. Let it happen in one flowing movement like a wave falling back into the ocean.

- After the exhalation there is a natural pause much like in the ocean when the waves seem to rest before they come back up. Don't hold the breath at either end; ocean waves do not stop at the crest, the pause is a natural part of the wave. Let the breath flow in a similar continuous pattern. Your mouth and your jaws stay relaxed as you visualize the wave filling you up from the bottom much like when you pour water into a container and the water fills the container from the bottom. Do not attempt to control the inhalation either. You don't have to pull in or push out the waves. As your belly relaxes into a full exhalation feel the inhalation follow on its own without effort. When you relax the belly and open the mouth then the breath just rushes in without effort.

This breath is very relaxing and invigorating. Start with a ten-minute practice (set a timer in case you drift off to sleep) and build up to half an hour.

# 5   Innocence and Imagination

"My daughter talks to cows, she doesn't need a stick," my father said to the men of our village.

Outraged, four men had cornered my father in the town square, "You cannot send a six-year-old to pasture ten cows without a stick!"

Innocent to the limitations of these men, my father lived outside of dogma and convention. From him I learned to sing to the cows and befriend them with a tender and loving voice. This approach was far more appealing to my sensitive, loving nature than swatting a wide-eyed heifer with a stick.

What is innocence? The ability to see, feel, hear, touch and experience what is happening *for what it is* in all its fullness without projecting pre-conceived notions and interpretations onto that fluid ever-changing reality. I did not see the cows as chattels; they were my friends. I loved the way they licked the salt off my hands with their sticky rough tongues. My father trusted my love for the cows. When I asked to take them up the mountain to pasture he said yes. Being able to control those big animals with my voice alone gave me a sense of competence and strength. Finally, I could do something my sister could not.

Like a baby who is open and innocent by nature the innocent face of Eve seeks a relationship with reality that is unencumbered. Her innocence saw no evil in tasting the forbidden fruit. The apple simply invited her and she accepted the invitation. She saw eating the fruit as another experience of fullness. The apple was not just an apple; it was a new experience, one that would reveal more about the world.

Innocent perception is a crucial skill in healing work as it allows a fresh, unconditioned perspective on human behavior. All behavior can be understood and unraveled if we look at it with non-judgmental eyes. From the perspective of Tantra yoga, reality is empty by nature. Enlightenment means having no argument with reality or with the multiplicity of all manner of experience that constantly saturates our perceptual systems. In the West, we habitually see through the lens of duality—good and evil, right and wrong. Innocent perception sees not an evil nature but habits of behavior with undesirable results. These behaviors are not signs of evil; they are a sign that the person is experiencing frustration and pain he or she does not know how to deal with in any other way. Is this evil or ignorance? To divide reality into good and evil is not

*"Enlightenment means*

*having no argument with reality"*

adequate. We must look thoroughly at what is happening.

When working within the framework of Tantra, specific breath and awareness practices catalyze and ignite love—the most powerful force in the human psyche. I teach clients to use all the energies of love that express uniquely through each of the seven chakras. A distinct vibration and potent source of healing, love expresses through each of the chakras in a specific way:

- first chakra—located in the subtle body in the area corresponding with the perineum, governs the earth element and the sense of smell; when this chakra is open and balanced you feel relaxed and safe

- second chakra—corresponds with the sex organs, governs the water element and the sense of taste; when open and balanced, you are aware of the pleasure of your erotic and creative energy

- third chakra—associated primarily with the solar plexus area, governs the fire element and the sense of sight; when open and balanced, you feel empowered to be the best you can be, have the inner will to achieve that and be competent and assertive without controlling others

- fourth chakra—the heart center, corresponds with the physical heart, governs the sense of touch and the element of air; when open and balanced allows you to feel unconditional love for yourself and for another, compassion for the difficulties of the human condition, and passion for giving and receiving love

- fifth chakra—the throat center, governs sense of hearing and is associated with space; when open and balanced this chakra facilitates speaking the truth clearly and being highly creative.

- sixth chakra—known as the third eye and located at the center of the forehead, governs intuition, sometimes called the "sixth sense" and is associated with light; when open and balanced can be clairvoyant, it allows you to observe life from a higher vantage point, and make decisions with greater ease and confidence

- seventh chakra—at the crown of the head, known as the thousand petal lotus; when open and balanced you experience transcendence, unity consciousness, and come to know the Self as one with cosmos and God/Goddess

Remember, that all chakras are perfectly spiritual; they are not higher or lower in terms of more or less spiritual. The Higher chakras have faster vibrations, shorter waves, and higher frequencies.

The lower chakras vibrate slower, have longer waves and are more dense.

Chakras are transformers of universal energy.

To better understand the nature of universal energy we can compare it to something we are all familiar with: electricity.

A high voltage electrical current would burn out a receiver that can only handle 110 volt, so too with Universal Energy.

Universal energy is a very high frequency and is stepped down to gradually lower frequencies through each chakra so it can be absorbed by the body .

Besides acting as transformers of energy, the chakras can also store energy, just as capacitors can store electricity and release it on demand.

Although the Chakra system does more than store energy, if we think of it in these terms, a man's ejaculation causes a sudden loss of energy when the stored vitality contained in the semen is spent.

Tantra teaches methods to fill up the system whenever it needs replenishing. Tantra never says what we should do but instead makes us aware of the consequences of our actions and offers a choice. Tantra offers tools to replenish the spent energy and teaches how to circulate the energy from the sex center through the whole system up to the crown chakra—many times, if desired—before ejaculating. This allows a man to stay in an energized state; an ejaculation does not shut down the system and cause a man to fall asleep leaving the woman alone. The couple can continue sharing and nurturing in many other ways: pillow talk, hugs, and more.

In Tantra, the sexual energy is stirred up with breathing and desire, then it is transformed into the energy contained in each Chakra, i.e. power, love, clear communication, intuition and connection with All that IS. This can continue for as long as you want. You can climb the mountain of ecstasy knowing that the higher you climb the better your orgasm is going to be. This high-octane orgasm is superior in quality and strength to an initial ejaculation that may or not be an orgasm at all. Men tell me that sometimes when they ejaculate too soon (a time frame that is different for everyone) they just feel a release of tension, but not the earth-shaking orgasm that they have when they sustain their lovemaking longer.

After a high octane orgasm men are usually not depleted because they have been charging their chakra system all along and can be present to enjoy the afterglow with their lover.

Or, better still, men can choose to have an earth-shaking body orgasm without ejaculation that leaves them fully satisfied and full of energy.

Another important fact to add is that the chakras are wheels that spin clockwise in the front and counterclockwise in the back. They take in universal energy from the back on the inhalation, then fill the body and send the overflow forward through their clockwise spinning action on the exhalation. Being conscious of this flow helps the practitioner place his or her intention on opening up the back to increase the intake of energy and then open up the front to send energy to our lover, having absorbed what we needed in our chakra capacitor.

Few people come to Tantra with their chakras open and balanced; most are either closed or open and unbalanced. In either case, they are functioning sub-optimally. For example, a person with a heart center that is too open can be 'co-dependant' and stay in an unhealthy relationship that does not serve him or her. When the heart center is closed or only partially open, a person cannot fully love and be loved. When our chakras are balanced, all these vibrations can be put to the service of healing. With these powerful forces, healing can take place much faster and go much deeper than through traditional talk therapy. When I start work with a client, I begin by tuning and clearing the energy of these primary chakras, thus strengthening the flow of vital energy along the central vertical axis of the body.

The vertical line is a profound theme in both Tango and Tantra. Tango stresses the vertical line that goes from the coccyx bone down to the core of the earth, up to the crown of the head and above to infinity and even beyond. The deeper you go into the earth the higher you can ascend.

There is no performance goal. Your goal is connection rising to the highest potential. This is not a co-dependant relationship like two invalids joined at the hip. This is union in ascension. While the feet constantly caress the ground to absorb the earth energy, the torso and the head are kept floating up. In the front of the chest, the heart is kept soft and open to the energy of the other. Each person is in total power in their own body and paradoxically in total surrender to each other into the full expression of the music.

This is a similar dynamic weaving of masculine and feminine energies as occurs in *yab-yum*, the highest of the tantric positions. In yab-yum position lovers face each other: the man sits in lotus position while the woman sits on his lap, her legs wrapped around his body with the toes of both her feet touching near his sacrum. This completes the energy circuits and enhances the connection. Both Tantra and Tango stress the vertical line to make the dance of love the highest expression of the Union of the human with the divine.

Teddy came to see me expressing a longing to connect fully with a woman. Those were not his exact words but I understood that what he was really missing was the ability to connect. He had tried several times to have a sexual relationship but he knew nothing about *intimacy*. He had never really seen himself fully. He avoided intimacy with women out of a fear that they might see something horrible and run away. He was afraid to take a real good look at himself. His greatest fear was that someone would see the sexual addiction he kept hidden under a tremendous burden of shame.

Teddy's sexual addiction was masturbation, which he had come to prefer over intercourse. He did not enjoy sex with women and was concerned that this was due to his preference for self-stimulation. Part of him wanted to give up trying to have a relationship with a woman altogether for he no longer wanted to feel like a failure. However his need to connect with the other sex was too strong to let him get away with avoidance. He did not know how to connect to a real being and his inner self, his unconditioned innocence, was reaching out for help.

Teddy had no idea how to be intimate, how to touch the body and the soul of a woman. He had not even been able to connect with himself that way. He used his sexuality to release tension; he never really made love to himself. He thought it strange to love yourself while doing something shameful like sex.

Obviously he had put sex in the category of shameful activity.

"Sex is something you do because it feels good and since it's bad then you do it in hiding," he said. What he had learned about sex early in life was not much different from what I had learned, only less dramatic. No one had told him that by touching himself he would put nails in Christ's body! The negative implant he had received was that sex is sinful unless you use it for procreation. And the last thing he wanted to do was make a child. Therefore shame and guilt were his only options with respect to sex.

Teddy never questioned this shame-based belief and never asked himself as I had, "Now, why would God make something that is so pleasurable and uplifting a sin?" Because he did not question this belief, the negative implant sent a deep root into his psyche. The pain of this old-world style of thinking brought him to a turning point and Teddy was open to learning how to love. Having experienced over and over again that shameful sex left him empty and deeply depressed, he'd finally had enough. It is often at these "Enough!" moments that we are ripe for change.

When I asked Teddy to tell me about his first experience of masturbation, he was surprised. Never had he imagined that he would experience being completely accepted once he revealed his *secret*. The innocence of my question allowed him to respond in kind—from the innocence of his unconditioned self. A trusting place emerged between us; the danger of being shamed no longer colored his view of himself.

He explained, "As a boy, I watched from my window as a beautiful woman in the house across the street undressed. As she slowly took off her clothes, she touched her breast and immediately got a strong erection. I remembered how the breast of my mother felt when I was an infant, remembered how loved I felt, and these memories together gave me an immediate and powerful ejaculation. In comparison to that, intercourse has always seemed pale."

As we explored further, Teddy came to see that he preferred masturbation because it allowed him to express his sexuality with a sense of childhood innocence where he had no responsibility to another. As a child, food and touch were provided for him and required no effort on his part. He felt no expectations pressuring him so he could relax and let go easily. The power of both his erection and ejaculation had to do with the complete void of expectation as to performance.

He did not know then that Tantra suggests no goal in sexual expression other than connection with another and the attainment of enlightened awareness. He was actually connecting with himself but in a childlike mode in which he need not give to another but simply receive pleasure. He was obviously now ready to explore his sexuality in an adult context and allow his sexuality to mature so as to involve another.

In the Pathwork Lecture[5], titled *The Forces of Love, Eros, and Sex,* Eva Pierrakos and The Guide address the maturing of our sexuality this way: "There is no such thing as a force, a principle, or an idea

---

[5] © *Eva Pierrakos and the Pathwork Foundation. See: www.pathwork.org*

that is in itself sinful whether sex or anything else. In the growing child who is naturally immature, the sex drive will first manifest selfishly. Only if and when the whole personality grows and matures harmoniously will sex become integrated with love.

Out of ignorance, humanity has long believed that sex as such is sinful. It was kept hidden and therefore this part of the personality could not grow up. Nothing that remains in hiding can grow... sex remains childlike and separate from love."

For Teddy, coming out of hiding and sharing his experience allowed him to heal the block of shame that had arrested his emotional development. As he felt washed clean by clear understanding, more of his adult self became engaged. He was released from the stranglehold of cultural projections that *sex is sinful* and returned to a state of natural innocence.

Innocence is the visible face of Eve that washes clean all the cultural imprints. Thus cleared, we come fully present in our power and vulnerability as man or woman. We are ready to experience the real truth of our Human/Divine experience.

Again, from Pierrakos channeling The Guide, we hear: "If people would realize—and they are beginning to do so increasingly—that the sex instinct is as natural and God-given as any other universal force and in itself not more sinful than any other existing force, they would then break this vicious circle and more human beings would let their sex drives mature and mingle with love – and with Eros, for that matter."

Sex has had a bad rap for many of us. Our loss of innocence in

*"Tantra suggests no goal in sexual expression
other than connection with another and the attainment of
enlightened awareness"*

this area is precisely what prevents our sexuality from being able to mature. Reclaiming that lost innocence opens the door so we can learn the best use of erotic/sexual energy.

Contrary to prevailing notions that sexuality is a power to be ashamed of and to be avoided or sublimated, sensual energy can help us grow in many ways. The physical experience is just the beginning. Beyond that, we can discover that fully embracing our sexuality as an innocent and powerful energy can allow us to connect on a soul level. When this merging happens we experience a state of unity with all that exists and gain access to a timeless space of bliss that is indescribable. How to use sensual energy as the fuel to reach spiritual orgasmic experiences is covered by Tantra, a scientific, spiritual, common sense—and at the same time esoteric—approach to life.

I did not know that flower arranging was a tantric art when I attended my first Tantra class. I arrived at the hotel where the class was being held in full possession of my natural curiosity and innocence. By then a working psychotherapist for ten years, I had taught yoga in both Italy and New York City, and had studied yoga with an Indian Guru whom I followed to India. When I read about the upcoming Tantra workshop I knew it would be the perfect next step for me.

I arrived early as is my habit. Jimmy was the first person I saw. He was draping colorful pieces of silk from columns in the large hotel conference room. The silk drapes immediately transformed the environment and I was immediately affected by Jimmy's natural grace.

When I saw him walk toward me with two vases and several bunches of wrapped flowers on a tray I asked if he wanted some help. He looked at me with appreciation; a tingling sensation moved through my body. I returned his admiring gaze appreciating his shiny, suntanned skin, and his well-muscled body.

This first exchange between us was sprinkled with such delight that I almost reached out to touch his perfectly shaved head, which shined as brilliantly as the candles he was lighting. Little did I know when he gave me a sip of his freshly squeezed carrot-ginger juice that this man would become Shiva embodied and my first real tantric lover. That juice was the most delicious juice that I ever tasted! Eros transformed the chemistry of that juice and would soon change the chemistry of my body as well.

With the innocence of a little girl who has never arranged flowers, I asked, "How do you want the flowers arranged?" Completely happy to serve alongside Jimmy in his task of setting up the room, I allowed him to direct me. As I watched him divide the flowers according to size, color and energy, I sensed the tremendous power of being with a man who consciously embraced Shakti, the universal energy of the feminine. Here was someone who stirred feelings in me as deep and as brilliant as my beloved teacher, Giuliana—only in a man's body!

Warm rivers of energy flowed through my veins making me almost dizzy. A powerful erotic energy began to envelop both of us. I knew from the look in his eye that Jimmy was feeling something similar. I felt the energy between us circulate, build, and move both inside and outside my body and his as though we were surrounded by a warm cocoon. I followed him everywhere. We turned on the light together while our lips touched and shivers of light coursed through our bodies. Anything we did together was magnetic and completely joyous.

Jimmy gave me my first taste of what it means to be with a man who consciously practices embodying Shiva, the masculine principle of the universe. Jimmy had achieved a level of integration where he could balance both Shiva and Shakti. Even before the workshop began, I was in an orgasmic state of discovery—innocence and curiosity mingling together—a really great space to discover tantric love.

During the workshop, the leader, Lori Star, asked the participants to pair up and sit facing each other. We touched each other with facial expressions, words, eyes, heart, and powerful feelings. Then we were guided to take turns to experience the tantric touch as both the Giver and the Receiver. As a giver, the goal was to give the touch being fully focused on the receiver with no expectations of being touched back. As a receiver the goal was to receive the touch staying connected only with the sensations of surrendering without focusing on giving back. To relax and receive fully is a great gift to the giver.

It was more challenging than I thought. For me it was easier to give. Jimmy and I took turns; his hands were perfect, soft yet strong. As breath merged with touch, I felt him reach in and caress the core of my being. The gap between our two bodies seemed to melt. I was inside and outside his hands—receiving all he was giving.

We became quite hot for each other as all the other energies were expressed and acknowledged. At this point the leader invited us to connect with the third eye. We were instructed to pull the energy we had generated up the Chakra system both with our intention and with a full breath that filled the whole body all the way up into the Crown Chakra. During the exhalation we then allowed the old air to leave the body while the charged particles of the life force contained in the breath were bathing all the chakras with renewed energy all the way down to the Root Chakra. Giving and receiving became one and the same at that point. We became a man-woman circle instead of two separate poles.

Tango invites this same phenomenon as the distinction between who's leading and who's following dissolves into the dance. The high art of relating—whether to a dance partner, a spouse, or someone you've just met on Match.com—challenges us to *blend our energy harmoniously with another.* Of course, there is no harmony without disharmony and some measure of discipline and learning goes into any art form. We may stumble and trip on one another at first but eventually we learn each other's dance steps—or not. Relationships live or die over our ability or inability to blend while remaining whole and intact as ourselves.

Countless relationships have died due to tainted perceptions of one another. An inability to forgive *and forget* plagues many a

*"The high art of relating—*

*whether to a dance partner, a spouse, or someone you've just met*

*on Match.com—challenges us*

*to blend our energy harmoniously with another"*

marriage. We come to expect *the same old same old* of each other and even fail to give each other the benefit of the doubt. This is where innocent perception becomes a great resource.

Next time you find yourself in a *locked-horns* type of situation with someone you love, choose to look and see if you aren't seeing that person through tainted eyes. Ask yourself, "Could it be that I have over-interpreted or second-guessed his or her actions or motives?" Try hitting the re-set button on your perception. Become open to not-knowing and innocent enough to really see the person as they are right now rather than rely on what comes from inside your mind. You might be surprised at how love grows when you relinquish a conditioned point of view.

### Lesson: Puja—A Tantric Ritual

This ritual is designed to bring out innocent perception and help you see the divinity in one another.

### Exercise:

- The woman stands or sits in front of her man and looks at him with a completely different eye; the eye that looks beyond personality and into the essence of who he is at the core.

- Both partners take a deep breath and bow to the other as a pure expression of Divinity; he an incarnation of God and she an incarnation of the Goddess.

- They bow and say the word, "Namaste," allowing the meaning of this salutation, "The God/goddess in me sees and honors the God/goddess in you," to adjust their seeing.

- The Goddess/Woman sees all that is pure, beautiful, passionate, loving, soft and strong, powerful, courageous, and real in her man.

- She gently flings open the doors of her heart and embraces this wonderful being who has the courage to love and endure all of what life on this plane involves.

- Now, the God/Man focuses on seeing the Goddess in his Woman.

- He sees all that is nurturing, safe, creative, soft and powerful, innocent, allowing, generous, open, and loving in her and rises to meet her in love.

- He allows a spiral of energy to rise from his sexual center into his heart and expresses that love by touching her heart Chakra gently.

- She then follows his lead and reaches out to touch his heart.

- Remain in this state of innocent seeing and refrain from talking. Your focus for these moments is to the soul level of your lover, not the personality. Complete the puja with the Yab-Yum tantric embrace, and allow yourselves to melt even further and become the Divine Couple. Shiva and Shakti exist as archetypal energies that will fill your lovemaking with new levels of meaning over time as you continue this practice.

**Lesson: Innocence in Tango**

If you go to a Milonga and observe couples dance, you will notice that no one seems to be looking at anyone else on the dance floor, thrilled as they are by the connection they are creating note by note with their partners. Tango encourages an innocent focus on each other; no comparison with others intrudes to distract the dancer's mind. Find a couple who looks very connected and in your imagination put yourself in their connection. Imagine you feel their connection in your body. Find another couple and notice how differently they connect. Become aware of the myriads of way people can connect.

Tango dancing is an exercise in acceptance of body appearance. In no way does the man judge the woman or the woman the man's appearance. Only the realness of their energy and their conscious effort to connect and dance is important.

Women can trust men's purity of intention in leading them in Tango. This trust is based on the safety that the Tango structure provides. Obviously, this takes time and practice, but making a commitment to grow in this direction is the first step.

**Exercise:**

Specific preliminary steps precede the actual visible movement part of the Argentine Tango. If you don't dance Tango yet, try it with someone you want to experiment with at home to get the feel for it.

1.  The man holds out his hand and invites the woman to dance with him.

2.  She nods and accepts the invitation and moves toward him.

3.  Man and Woman stand in front of each other and breathe to connect their energies.

4.  He reaches his left arm around her upper back and she settles into his embrace adjusting her left arm on his upper back near his neck.

5.  On the right side of the woman's body they hold hands, relaxing the arms and shoulders.

6.  The woman engages her belly muscles to support her balance and allows the front of her heart Chakra to melt into the man. Again, both the male and the female elements play a role in the Tango hug.

7.  They take time to feel each other's change of weight almost imperceptibly.

8.  Only after they both know on what foot the body's weight is do they take the first step to start the actual moving dance.

# 6 Honesty and Sacred Communion

One day when I was about six, I saw a little boy from my village urinate while standing near a tree. Ever curious, I wanted to see how he did this; I had to bend my knees to pee! How did he accomplish this marvelous act?

When next I saw Vito, I invited him to come over and play. We'd collected a large pile of hay on the farm and when he arrived the two of us threw ourselves onto the hay pile, laughing and poking and playing around. The hay was warm and scratchy but we did not care. When I asked, "Can I see where you pee from?" he was more than happy to show me. Surprised to see this little thing hanging out of his body, I touched it. He smiled.

"It's so soft," I said.

"Can I see where you pee from?" he asked.

I, too, was happy to show him.

At that moment, my sister walked out from behind the barn with a basket full of freshly laundered clothes. She walked toward the clothesline and heard us giggling in the haystack. Once she came around to where she could see us she immediately began to scold me, "Bad girl! Stop that!"

Vito scurried off as my sister berated, "You're bad, bad, bad."

Unsure as to what I had done wrong, I succumbed to my sister's elder-child authority and took on her shame-based view. The dynamic of shame has so strong a pull that even in our innocence we respond with embarrassment to a strong projection of "Bad!" such as the one my sister lobbed in my direction that day.

"Don't tell mom!" I begged, having swallowed her shame like the bitter pill it was.

My sister agreed not to tell mom and offered a *bribe* in exchange for her silence. "I won't tell but you have to do some of my chores." This continued for almost a year until I grew into thinking for myself. Eventually, I came to realize that what I'd done had not hurt anyone. I had been curious and that was no sin. *Let mother know*, I thought, now willing to take the consequences directly rather than hide out of shame. And so, I told my sister "Go ahead and tell mom if you want! And you can sweep the porch yourself!"

But my sister did not tell our mother. I had a normal load of chores again and I felt lighter and stronger.

This was an early and potent lesson about honesty. It showed me that if I had the courage to be honest I would gain access to personal power. Standing up to my sister that day taught me a very basic lesson about human interaction and that telling the truth made me feel strong.

This incident served as a counter-point to a prevalent attitude in our village that it was stupid to be honest. According to this view, which is still prevalent in many corners of the world, the honest person is at a distinct disadvantage because telling the truth gives others an opening to take advantage of his or her vulnerability. Honesty is associated with vulnerability rather than strength. In the tantric view, vulnerability and strength are two sides of one coin. One cannot have strength without vulnerability. The two are wed by their very nature. The juxtaposition of two seemingly opposite forces is the very tension that makes life interesting. And it is this same tension that propels our growth and evolution.

At age of thirteen, this tension catapulted me into a new life.

I always adored the first breath of spring. All the wild flowers and tulips were coming into bloom and I was finally free to take off the scratchy thick stockings we had to wear all winter high in the Alps. My naked legs delighted at the feel of the breeze and the direct touch of the fabric of my dress.

One day while pasturing the cows in the woods, I decided to collect some flowers to put on the altar of Mary. It being May—the month dedicated to Mary—I wanted to express my great love for her. As I picked a colorful bouquet of wild violets, blue forget-me-nots, and wild white lilies, a great surge of energy flowed through my body. When I was done, I sat down and took stock of the cows pasturing peacefully on the hillside.

My older brother was coming up the mountain from the ridge below. As I looked a second time, I noticed a flask of Chianti in his hand. As he drew nearer I saw that the flask was half empty. He was red in the face and charged with strange energy. Immediately, I knew something was awry and began to feel scared. I started to sing softly to push away my fear but my voice became stuck in my throat as he approached. He came toward me and, without a word, pushed me to the ground. Hurt by the rough stones under my body, I squealed and tried to scramble away. He ignored my protest and pushed me beneath him pulling a very swollen sex organ out of his pants. This was only the second penis I had ever seen and it looked nothing like the one Vito had shown me in the hay. This one was huge and scary looking. My brother tore off my underpants and pushed himself into me. It hurt and burned as he pushed in and out many times. The smell of wine on his breath made me nauseous, but strangely enough, I started to feel a pleasurable sensation along with the pain. This confused me deeply. Then, as suddenly as he'd come upon me, he stopped, pulled himself out of me and ran down the mountain without saying a word.

Shocked and confused, I picked myself up and began to rub the soreness in my back from being pushed onto the uneven rocky ground. When I saw the blood around my vagina I began to cry, praying aloud to Mother Mary, "What just happened? I do not understand... Please help me!"

I dared not leave the cows even in my distress and brought them down the mountain, crying all the way. Once I reached the farm, I ran to my mother, sobbing. I knew that my father would not be any help; he had long since taken refuge in a world all his own. His ability to deal with human interactions was quite limited. I knew this situation was way out of his range.

When I told my mother what had happened her mouth dropped open. I will never forget the horrified look on her face as her eyes grew wide and bulged out of her head. She said not one word and all but froze. She made no move to hug me or offer solace. This left me even more hurt and confused. "Was it my fault?" This sneaky doubt crept in despite my certainty that I was innocent. The schism between these two thoughts—*It's my fault*, and, *I'm innocent*—was like a painful boil that would not go away for many years to come.

Now I understand that the shock of this news caused my mother to push what I'd told her out of her mind and into her subconscious. Unable to accept that this could happen to her—a woman who got up every day at 5 a.m. to go to mass in the nearby convent—caused her mind to simply disassociate from what I had said.

I could not slip into denial with her, however. Honesty was and is my essential nature; I *had* to tell the truth. In this sense, I was still innocent. I had not learned to lie—not even to myself. When we are innocent we are naturally honest because we don't distort or deny our experience. We simply observe and relate things as they are. Children are our greatest teachers on this score. Before they get the

*"When we are innocent we are naturally honest because we don't distort or deny our experience. We simply observe and relate things as they are"*

opposite lesson from the so-called grown-ups around them and learn to manipulate situations to get what they want, children are fully honest. They feel their emotions intensely. When they are happy, they giggle and smile. When they are hungry or hurt, they scream. Slowly, over time, they learn to mask what they feel to change the outer expression in order to change the outcome. Thus, they prepare the soil in their mind for the prickly plant known as lying. Like a cactus that uses its needles to protect itself, lies are almost always an attempt to avoid pain or rejection of some sort.

As we know, lies may help us avoid unpleasant consequences in the short run but they undermine relationships in the long run. Honesty is the hidden face of Eve that, once unveiled, allows all the other hidden faces to shine their brilliant light into the open.

We make so much more progress when we stop thinking in terms of good and bad behavior and simply ask ourselves to be honest. As Rumi said in the C. Barks translation: "Out beyond all ideas of right doing and wrong doing there is a field. I'll meet you there."

Honesty is the path into that field.

In the movie, *Kama Sutra,* the beautiful slave-girl, Maya, learns about the rules of love and the nature of honesty and deceit. Upset by an unsavory encounter with her one-time lover, the king, Maya retreats to the home of Rosa Devi, her confidante and mentor in the arts of love. She listens to Rosa Devi's wise counsel, "Some men can be like animals, but it is not all men. Since when is woman simply a helpless animal? Just like men we are awake and filled with longing. Passion remains the spirit behind existence, Maya, nothing will ever change that. It's how we *use* our passion that's of essence. Now, we must listen to what the Kama Sutra teaches—the true union between man and woman can take us beyond this animal lust into total trust and merging with the other. Each becomes both; imagine such bliss."

For a tantric couple, honesty is both cornerstone and sharpening-stone of the relationship. Honesty is the quality that ripens romance and allows it to grow in trust and forge a deeper intimacy between them.

Romance and intimacy are very different. Romance is largely a matter of personality whereas intimacy involves character.

Chemistry, charm, and sexual attraction lure us into romance where the social self plays with somebody else's social self. We are entranced by romance candlelight dinners, exotic honeymoons, and luxurious bubble baths. But when the romantic bubble pops—who is the person next to you?

Intimacy, on the other hand, both sharpens and draws out our deeper character. We relinquish even the subtlest pretense and reveal our authentic self. This allows us to bond with another essence-to-essence and express our soul's deepest longing.

The tantric couple makes a commitment to keep their love fresh by scheduling special times for lovemaking at least once a week. In the beginning phase a relationship is new and exciting. Chemistry carries us over any rough spots and we tend to see only what is good in our partner. After a couple years we seem to know all about our partner. We've made love in all imaginable positions in every room in the house. Boredom starts to creep in. To avoid slipping into complacency over time we must venture into deeper realms of emotion, psyche, and spirit. Setting aside time for erotic play is essential. Some couples commit to a short time of physical connection once a day even if for only ten minutes. The intention is to nurture and care for one another without a specific goal around sex. As a ritual practice this keeps the heart open. Problems are more easily resolved when the heart space between two is regularly fed with simple presence.

Sharon and Eric committed to this practice when they reconciled after a three-month trial separation. Between the day-to-day busyness of running two businesses and raising their two-year old they had drifted quite far apart. Each little problem contributed to the gap between them until they could hardly speak to one another. During their time apart, Sharon, who is a yoga teacher by profession, took a weekend class with me. When she moved back home to live with her husband they committed to one simple practice—sitting together facing each other for ten minutes every morning. Those ten minutes could be spent eye-gazing, hugging, kissing, breathing together, or even crying. Their only rule is: no talking. They have maintained this practice for three years now and their marriage is on solid ground.

## Lesson: Can this person go the distance?

The following questions, answered honestly, will help you reflect on whether or not the one you love can go the distance and journey through romance into intimacy with you. (Note: you might do well to ask these questions of yourself first.)

1. Has your sweetheart confessed to any immoral behavior like cheating, stealing, lying, excessively aggressive behavior, or violence? If so, does he/she reflect on what happened and demonstrate both a desire and the motivation to change?

2. Does your lover have any addictions like drinking, gambling, or shopping? Is he or she working toward change or just promising to do so?

3. Does he or she have many lasting friendships? Just a few? None to speak of?

4. Is your loved one solution-oriented or prefers to complain about innumerable conflicts with others?

5. Does he or she value personal growth and demonstrate this by being able to problem-solve when your respective grievances arise? Or does he/she simply tell you what you want to hear to make the problem *go away* while still being unresolved?

6. Does your loved one truly value open communication and know how to listen? When you are upset or need to be nurtured, does he or she deal with it directly or are you noticing a tendency to shut down, attack, or speak in a condescending manner?

*"Couples who tend to stay together know how to fight so that each person gets to win"*

7.  Is your loved one willing to practice sitting still together just to breathe and allow your minds to grow quiet and your bodies experience a warm flow of energy?

It's not how well you get along in a relationship that really matters; it's how well you hear each other's needs and come to a mutually agreeable solution to meet them. Couples who tend to stay together know how to fight so that each person gets to win. A couple is strong when they know how to cope with their weakest moments successfully.

## Lesson on Communication

Good communication is the most important ingredient in the relationship soup. Great sex can be maintained when couples keep nothing hidden from each other—nothing disturbing or negative and nothing exhilarating and positive. They are both important. I call it radical honesty sweetened by compassion with the intention of letting your partner know **the real you in each moment** of your togetherness. Honesty is the greatest aphrodisiac because it allows us to come from newness and vulnerability.

The following communication model is loosely based on Marshal's Rosenberg's model of *Non-Violent Communication*, which has inspired me greatly. I strongly recommend his book by that title.

## Exercise:

This practice can help you deal with conflicts and share matters of concern in a positive way before they escalate into major problems.

Person A: There is something I would like to tell you so I can deepen my love for you.

Person B: Please tell me

A: I have been avoiding sex because I'm feeling resentful about some of your behavior and wanted to punish you.

B: Thank you for telling me that. Is there more you want to tell me?

A: Yes, I just realize that I am punishing myself as well and I no longer want to do it. I would feel that you consider my feelings if you called me when you know you are going to be late for dinner.

B: I will do it.

A: How do you feel knowing that I wanted to punish you?

B: I feel happy that you told me. I noticed you were avoiding making love to me and that confused me because I could not imagine the reason for it. Now that you have told me I feel relieved. You have made a conscious decision to tell me and that inspired me to give you what makes you feel loved. I like how this honesty game works. May I invite you to tell me if something is bothering you as soon as you notice?

A: Yes.

# 7   Courage: The Vital Life Force

Each of us sees the world in a manner that is consistent with how our psyche is composed. If we believe that life is pain then our psyche will attract painful experiences or interpret our experience as painful in order to be consistent. While the soul longs for newness and truth in the moment, the mind seeks to repeat what it knows. Confusion is an uncomfortable experience psychologically speaking. Remaining consistent with our identity—the beliefs, self-concept, and points of view we hold on to as *who I am*—allow us to avoid the discomfort of change. The psyche naturally tends to create clarity by vibrating at a level that attracts the very circumstance that will prove its point of view.

This conundrum has led more than one seeker of truth to ask the question, "Would I rather be right or happy?" Whenever I had to choose between the two, *my* answer has always been, "I'd much rather be happy than right."

We grow more rapidly when we take full responsibility for our actions and reactions. Failing to do so we miss the hidden play of the subconscious mind. This peculiar blindness, which is not at all uncommon, can convince us we are victims of other people or the world at large. Displacing responsibility and blaming circumstances or other people for our discontent keeps us from growing.

Looking into our own mind and emotions to decipher the beliefs and attitudes that attracted the undesirable circumstance can bring us to a place of self-knowledge and understanding. Such an epiphany has the power to enlighten our behavior and attitude and bring our functioning to a higher level. This is the deeper meaning of the word *empowerment*.

Gandhi believed that when we live our truth we might have to let go of being consistent. Living our truth includes going through the discomfort of updating our reality map to fit the truth of the moment. Whether or not happiness is an inalienable right or not seems a moot point. Better to think of happiness as a choice. Only then can unhappiness be viewed from a useful perspective. When unhappiness surfaces then a self-responsible individual looks to see what limiting beliefs are attracting the unhappiness and chooses to do the inner work necessary to bring about a shift.

At a certain point in my life I decided to prove to myself that life could be more about joy and gratitude than anger and frustration. After acknowledging the background thoughts that were

*"Living our truth includes going through
the discomfort of updating our reality map
to fit the truth of the moment"*

keeping joy from expressing in my life and transforming them into joy-attracting thoughts, I came up with what seems a simple declaration: "I am now choosing to live my life in joy. I am in charge of my reactions. I am grateful for the blessings of each day."

As soon as I declared this, however, my body had a strange reaction. Fear gripped me in my gut and my breath became shallow. Would I become a Pollyanna and put myself at risk? Images appeared in my mind of an air-headed cricket who plays all summer long instead of working to put away food for the winter like the industrious little ants. In my mind's eye I saw the cricket begging the ants for food. My shoulders tightened up at this image and I noticed myself all but holding my shallow breath. Everything in me—my nervous system, my musculature, my endocrine glands, my thought patterns and emotions—had all been conditioned to work, work, work, and to reaffirm at every turn that life is hard and "a valley of tears." It takes a great deal of courage to feel the fear of changing any belief that has served us and jump into the unknown with another belief that has not proven its efficacy yet. And even after we decide mentally to try out a more positive belief, it still takes quite some time to integrate it on a cellular level. This new approach is by no means automatic and I still have to consciously make the shift at times.

*The good news is that the more we exercise conscious choice, the faster we can integrate the new direction.*

I think of these revisions in our basic way of being as *new belief implants.* To install a new program into a computer is easy because the computer has no emotional attachment to the old program. We need to really be actively *installing* the new programs several times before they're accepted on a cellular level. Neurolinguistic studies confirm that it takes 21 consecutive days to make a new groove in the brain and retrain the nervous system to act in a different way.

A great program is: "I find joy in everything I do."

The neural groove of old beliefs, being deeper, often kicks up the old way of seeing and reacting to life. Old beliefs may even re-emerge with powerful force.

*Uncomfortable feelings are a signal to pay attention and ask: "What groove have I fallen into now?"*

Emotions are energy in motion. What's more, emotions are usually caused by a thought we hold. The more we honor emotions without becoming their slave, the more our energy can increase. Once emotional energy is stirred up we end up consuming tremendous amounts of energy by either acting out the emotions dramatically or by keeping them blocked and suppressed. To get an idea just how much energy is involved in suppressing emotions, imagine squeezing something in your hand you don't want anyone to see. Go ahead, squeeze tight, and keep squeezing for ten minutes or longer. Notice how tired those hand muscles are and imagine how tired they will be after a full day of holding on. Yet many of us keep emotions suppressed for years.

The stuffed feelings lodge in our stomach, our sex center, or our throat. Through deep circular breathing, those emotions get stirred up—consciously and intentionally this time—allowing us to make a different choice and release the energy that goes into holding on.

*Deep, conscious, circular breathing is a great help in shifting from old patterns to the more life-affirming grooves.*

As a student of Carl Jung's psychotherapeutic approach, I was heartened to find confirmation for what I had discovered along these lines. Jung says that the psyche creates the way we see the world. Further, he reminds us that the word apocalypse means, "the unveiling of what has been hidden."

In apocalyptic times like ours, the light of Spirit begins to reveal what has been kept behind the veil of ignorance, misperception, or in some cases, outright deception. For some, that process is very painful, especially when the light reveals material that is so close to home that it threatens our very view of who we are. Such revelations require a lot of inner work and radical honesty as the unconscious *stuff* that we have blocked out of awareness returns to our conscious experience. This is a powerful way to become fully self-responsible.

*The hidden face of Eve I am calling Courage has the strength and wisdom to take up this course of radical honesty and self-awareness.*
She also has the courage to show compassion for people who are yet unaware of the power of their subconscious process. Condemnation of others ends as she expands her heart to embrace the human condition with total compassion. Even her own moments of forgetting are met with understanding. Whatever happens in the flow of life, she adopts an attitude of simple interest and relinquishes any tendency to judge. She is excited about being

*"When you know yourself as simple awareness then you know everyone's essence.*

*You can finally open your heart and simply be love"*

able to see through the illusion of the mind to look directly at what's happening and simply be aware. Joy comes with this courageous act. When you know yourself as simple awareness then you know everyone's essence. You can finally open your heart and simply be love. This is the deepest act of courage: to love in the face of any obstacle.

In *The Book of Secrets*, Osho says that when we really love our ego ceases to exist. Love means letting go of the illusion of security. When we love we don't know what will happen the next moment. We love because to do so fulfills our soul, not for what we will receive in return. Love knows no guarantee. We love knowing that the person we love could leave or die any day. When we love we risk tremendous loss and pain and yet we choose to love with our whole being.

David Schnarch, Ph.D., author of *Constructing the Sexual Crucible*, (Norton Professional Books, 1991) says this about why a good marriage will break your heart: "Love is not for the weak…In a long term marriage, one partner will bury the other. Marriage is a people growing machine; it stretches you to the point where you can embrace the process of Life and love on their own terms. Like intense intimacy and eroticism, real love is not for kids. It's for adults only."

Wilhelm Reich, father of the mind-body movement, began one of the most significant trends in psychology. Reich believed that every mental disease stems from lack of love. If we take this to be true then perhaps all such diseases can be healed by love. Agnes

Sanford, another early holistic thinker and famous healer in the early part of the twentieth century, identified love as the most powerful healing force of all. In her classic book, *Healing Light,* she speaks of love as, "...a powerful, radiant, and life-giving emotion, charged with healing power both to the one who learns to love and to the one who is loved."

Love requires courage. When we love we stretch beyond the self-protective limits of our known self and move toward another. And letting go of your protective limits takes courage.

Love is a gift of life we give ourselves out of that act of courage. And love happens only in the moment. We move out of the present when we ask, "How will it be to love this person in the future?" The very thought of the future lifts us out of the moment of bliss. Imagination then takes over and one or more scenarios—often scripted by our unconscious fears—come forward to distract the mind and intrude on the moment of bliss. On a subtle level, our vital energy leaves the heart center and jumps up to fuel the planning and strategizing activities of the mind.

In less than a heartbeat, love's bliss gives way to mental activity and we find ourselves making a project out of holding onto the person and the experience. This is especially so if the experience brings pleasure. The mind says, "No future? What?" and begins to weave a subtle panic that pulls us out of the moment.

*Society constantly encourages us to build and plan a better future; more wealth, more success, more accomplishments – these we are told, ought to be our primary aims.*

Does this mean we have to choose between love and security?

Christ helps us solve this dilemma with a simple sentence: "Be in the world but not of the world." Love requires the courage to be in the world, open-hearted and willing to accept what comes. Being in the world but not of the world does not mean being inept and doing nothing. Rather, this scripture suggests that we infuse our doing with love and genuine soul expression. This type of *doing* is free of tension because we do out of love, not obligation or expectation of a specific return.

Jennifer and David came to see me. As is my practice when working with couples, I asked them to answer some questions individually before they saw me together. David felt the relationship was on the verge of ending because Jennifer had suddenly stopped making love to him without explanation. He suspected she had found someone else. They had been married for two years and previously enjoyed a fantastic sex life. How could she close the door out of the blue? He'd had it. Ostensibly, he was coming to see me because she insisted; however, I sensed he had a deep desire to understand his wife.

When I saw Jennifer individually, she said that she never experienced a real orgasm with David. The trouble began when a girlfriend told her about the incredible extended orgasms she was experiencing with her husband. Seeing how radiant and happy her friend was, Jennifer decided she no longer wanted to miss out on this aspect of life. She loved her husband but felt ashamed of having faked her orgasms throughout their relationship. She asked me to advise her how to save her marriage without telling her husband the painful truth. Aside from David's sexual approach, she loved being with him. She simply had not been able to tell him the truth for fear of hurting his feelings.

Clearly, David and Jennifer were faced with a number of obstacles to the success of their marriage. The most obvious problem was a lack of communication with underlying issues stemming from a lack of real presence, and a lack of trust.

*Real love cannot grow without trust.*

Another challenge was Jennifer feeling responsible for David's feelings and David's belief that someone else could *make him* feel a certain way.

I invited David to come in for an individual session as well. He explained that his initial attraction to Jennifer was due in large measure to the fact that she bore a strong resemblance to his favorite porn star. This particular actress, David reported, always screamed when she reached orgasm and enjoyed being *thoroughly pounded.*

"Ah, how I always wished I could meet a woman like that," David said, "but a good woman, not a porn star. A woman who would make me feel like a real man."

David met Jennifer in his early twenties. "She was perfect," he said, "shy, good-looking, long blond hair, large, shapely breasts. She was a bit distant but I liked that. I thought if I could get her to fall in love with me I would really feel good."

So he started wooing Jennifer. He invited her to dine at luxurious restaurants and took her to the opera and ballet. He had a hunch she really liked that and he was right. She *fell in love*.

Separately, Jennifer confessed that she had fallen in love with an idea.

"I had this idea in my head that I would have a great life with him because he would take me to wonderful places. He offered the security I wanted. If I grew tired of working as a court stenographer, I could stop and have a nice life."

David explained that the first time he made love to Jennifer he wanted to marry her. "She made the same screaming sounds the porn star did and we looked so good together people would turn around and look at us on the street."

Clearly, both Jennifer and David were confused about love. When I asked David if he had ever loved anyone before Jennifer, he said, "No." When I asked about the relationship between his parents he explained that his parents were never affectionate in his presence. Further exploration revealed that David had never seen two people in love except for in a romantic movie. As a young man, he'd begun avoiding women because they often became "clingy" around him and seemed primarily interested in his wealth. He had formed the belief that women were only after his money. When he met Jennifer, she seemed different. "She did not cling to me," he said, citing this as another reason he allowed himself to fall in love.

During Jennifer's individual session, I learned that her parents and her brother had constantly warned her that, "women who throw their sexuality around end up poor and alone or with some loser." They often pointed out women who had failed to *marry well*, providing ample fuel for her growing fear that this could happen to her. Jennifer was very impressionable and, having grown up in a poor family, was frightened of continued poverty. So she vowed to herself that she would keep her sexuality under lock and key until she knew that the man was in love with her and wanted to get married.

These two young people were suffering the consequences of a *dangerous game: using sex to catch a partner* instead of to express love. Jennifer was taught to use sex as a tool to catch a man, rather than to celebrate life. When security is prized over love in a marriage, security wins.

Would this couple have the courage to say the truth to each other?

David and Jennifer had married young before either had come to a mature understanding of love; each had been drawn to the other on the basis of personal needs. Entering the great adventure of transcending the small self was not on their agenda but the pain they were experiencing was an invitation to grow in this direction. In their individual sessions, each took a giant step toward self-acknowledgement — a basic requirement for mature love. Together, they embraced the challenge of moving toward real love which meant setting their old agendas aside.

After a series of sessions, both separate and together, each started to get clear about their real desires and needs. As each slowly came down out of their head and into their real feelings, both felt a growing desire to love and be loved. The agenda of the small self gave way in each and a larger, shared vision of a life devoted to the other began to emerge.

Both David and Jennifer found the courage to step through the all-too-human resistance to seeing and speaking the naked truth. When Jennifer told the truth about faking her orgasms, David looked utterly aghast at first. Slowly, he brought himself around and let her finish speaking. In turn, David admitted that he'd been so involved in his fantasies of the porn star that he barely saw Jennifer as a real woman.

"I never even noticed how you were feeling," he said. Tears began to fill his eyes but David forced them back.

Jennifer could not hold back her tears; they flowed down onto her purple shirt. David told Jennifer that he was ready to learn how to be present with her. He wanted to help her heal from the negative sexual imprinting she had received.

"It might not be easy but you're worth it," he said. So much real caring filled that room as he said this Jennifer's heart flew open. I watched the spontaneous movement of love as they moved toward one another and shared the first real embrace of their life together. Watching their bodies, I could tell that they had broken completely new ground; neither of them had breathed that deeply and in such a relaxed manner in my presence before. I knew they had taken the first steps on the path of learning to love deeply.

Revealing these painful truths to each other required heroic strength of David and Jennifer. But soul strength they found; the revelation was the most important step this couple could have taken toward developing a real relationship. This is another secret of real love—we cannot really be in a relationship unless we are willing to let it go. David and Jennifer both took the risk of losing the other by revealing a shameful part of themselves, and both of them won.

## Lesson: Re-write your contract

Many of us had a less than perfect childhood and many of us—when the pain we felt as children seemed overwhelming—coped with it by making a contract with ourselves. The silent contract was made to cope with the situation at hand. It was powerful because it was made in a state of high energy and we made it to go on with life. So both the pain and the silent contract we made with ourselves got suppressed and we did not notice that we started living by that contract. An important part of self-awareness is to discover the contract and change it. This takes courage.

For instance, a boy who witnesses violence done by his father to his mother or siblings or who is himself the recipient of this violence might decide that he will never be like his father. This conclusion made at this powerful emotional point in his life goes deep into his psyche and becomes the contract by which he lives his life. Since as a child he might not have different family models he might also conclude that he would rather be like his mother who was more loving and not violent. However, so early in life he does not see that she does not stand up for what is right because she is afraid. And the boy makes an unconscious contract with himself: "I will never be like my father!" He will live by this contract until he discovers that there are other choices and that who he came to this life to be is perhaps completely different from his father and his mother.

# 8   Trust: A Full Embrace of Life

Part collie and part wolf, Pippo was always my favorite and most faithful childhood companion. We shared everything. Pippo ate my food, slept on my bed, and listened with keen canine attention to all the troubles bouncing about in my pre-adolescent head. Then, when I was twelve, Pippo ate a poisoned morsel of food. A man from our village had set the poison out in an attempt to kill a fox that was pilfering his chickens. For several hours that dragged on like days, I watched and tried to calm my beloved pet as he writhed in pain. From the look in his eyes I knew my dog was scared, as was I. Feeling sure he could fight the poison, I would not—could not— allow myself to think that he might die. And yet, after awhile, I noticed the look in Pippo's eyes change; he was no longer afraid. A calm sadness filled his eyes and his look seemed to implore me to accept his last good-bye. I nodded and caressed him, pouring all the love I felt for him through my hands into his body. We both understood what had to happen. His look became more and more relaxed until he finally took his last breath.

What Pippo taught me that day was the essence of trust. In the course of a brief morning I went from total fear and refusal to accept the inevitable to total understanding, acceptance and deep trust. All because of a wolf-collie's imploring look and the knowing that the love my dog and I had shared would never die.

Pippo's death brought me a moment of enlightenment. At that moment I understood that death is part of life. I was not aware then of how this event had begun to forge a deeper trust in life with the recognition of both the grace and inevitability of death. Grace, because death came to relieve my beloved Pippo from unbearable pain, and inevitability because the body is made of elements that naturally decompose. I have been in many dangerous situations that stirred up fear in me in the years since, and referring back to Pippo's death has always helped me reestablish trust. Living with an awareness of the inevitability of death gives us the courage to live fully.

Trust does not always come that easy, however. Fear can readily overtake us in challenging situations. At certain moments, life can become a maze poisoned by fear. Fear kept in the maze of the unconscious always deteriorates into a poison that kills us slowly over time often taking much longer to bring about our demise than the few hours it took for Pippo to die.

Of all the hidden faces of Eve, trust may well be the most difficult

*"Living with an awareness of the inevitability of death gives us the courage to live fully"*

to master. The primary block to trust is fear—an emotion that is deeply linked with survival. We need to distinguish between realistic fear and fear that comes from projection and imagination. Essential to our survival, for example, is a healthy fear of crossing the street when a car approaches at great speed. We just need to observe what happens and we know. Fear that poisons has a different source and purpose. Unhealthy fear grows out of projection and negative thought patterns that keep us from fully entering into life.

A balanced root chakra is essential for building a foundation of deep trust—trust in self, trust in others when appropriate, and trust in life. Energetically, root chakra issues are related to survival and yet imbalances and unaddressed issues at this level can make even minor slights seem like major threats. When trust is absent and old insecurities take over, we become *tight-assed*, literally tightening up our anal sphincters. We are afraid of opening up and giving of ourselves. This also manifests as *cold feet*—literally and symbolically. Both conditions cut us off from our vital connection with the earth. We block the spiraling movement of trust—that subtle force field that continually flows between the root chakra and terra firma to keep us safe and supported.

This energetic link with the earth can be discerned and felt by students of tai chi who use it to ground themselves when facing an opponent. In a relaxed and focused manner, the tai chi practitioner grounds him or herself, rooting into the earth. This creates a base of balance that cannot be readily moved.

The person who is afraid, on the other hand, holds his body in

*"The primary block to trust is fear—*
*an emotion that is deeply linked with survival"*

*"Trust can also manifest instinctively as an inner movement,*

*an impulse to make a major change"*

rigid stance that literally clips him at the knees (if not higher) and cuts him off from the earth as well as the fullness of his breath. In this stance, he can be thrown off balance with a slight push.

Trust can also manifest instinctively as an inner movement, an impulse to make a major change.

My first experience of being compelled by this type of life-changing soul-force breaking through into consciousness occurred when I was thirteen. After my brother raped me, a deep knowing that I must leave my family came so clearly I could not ignore it. "This is not where I'm supposed to be. I have no freedom to express myself and I don't feel safe in my home." This truth was so powerful, and the urge to make a change so strong, I dared an unprecedented act of courage and walked away from the only home I had ever known. The message came right through my bones but my legs were trembling. "Run away from home" is a figure of speech that did not apply at all. As I crossed the field toward the road out of town, I kept stopping to feel my feet sink into the grass. I guess you could say I walk-stop-sink, walk-stop-sink-ed away from home. With a heavy heart, I left my family and all the people I loved behind. By far one of the hardest decisions I ever had to make, this bold move taught me to trust the unknown. I walked all the way to the main road and continued walking until a car stopped.

Where did the knowledge that I must leave home come from? How did I know that "something better out there somewhere" was waiting for me? I had no knowledge of chakras and yet I listened to the infinite knowing that is always available. Trusting that inner knowing felt natural.

*Esoteric knowledge is not a prerequisite for receiving the inspiration to do what needs to be done.*

When a middle-aged man stopped at the side of the road to pick me up, my instinct told me I could trust him. I'd heard the horror stories of girls who'd been picked up hitchhiking and been killed and yet I knew that I could tell this man the truth. He asked where I was going and when I said, "I don't know," he knew he had a runaway on his hands. His genuine interest and concern were so tangible in the air between us that I told him the entire story of what had happened. This created even more trust.

Over the course of a day, I learned more about trust from this total stranger than I had learned in thirteen years from the family I left behind. He became a great benefactor and even went so far as to find me a new home and family once we crossed the border into Germany. How did I know to trust him? The signal came from my body. I felt relaxed and naturally began breathing deeply in the presence of such a *trustworthy* man. Around my mother and siblings I was always tense and on guard—I could rarely make a move without feeling afraid of doing it *wrong*.

*Those of us with this kind of tense early conditioning are vulnerable to the subtle fears that can poison relationships by pulling us out of the present moment—the only place where love can arise and be.*

Eddie and Cindy had been dating for a year but Eddie was not yet ready to commit to marriage. Age 35, Cindy's biological clock was ticking so fast she felt tense all the time. Lost in her own fear-maze, she was convinced her chances of becoming a mother were under serious threat if she waited much longer to marry. She started to become forceful and threatened to leave Eddie if he did not propose marriage within in the next 3 months. Each time she reminded him of this he pulled away more. Her forceful insistence—a common pattern Eva Pierrakos calls *the forcing current*—worked against the end she hoped to achieve. She called me in desperation sounding like a drowning woman reaching out for someone to save her.

Through our work together, Cindy began to see how the forcing current and her fear were causing her to become rigid rather than flexible and creative. She was able to work with me intensely, throwing herself into body centered therapy, yoga and tantric practice, and deep breathing to release the tight blocks of tension. As the inner pressure released she was able to lighten up on Eddie. Her loving nature re-emerged and she began to trust the love between them. He asked her to marry him two months later.

Acting out of inner tension often brings unpleasant consequences. If you want to be free to choose well you have first to unblock the tensions that scream out: "I want what I want right now!" Forcefully going for what we want is not the smartest path. You catch more flies with honey than with a swat.

To learn to trust we must deal with the immature ego. This takes keen awareness of the ego as it tends to nudge us to give up when situations become difficult or unpleasant. The ego also discourages trying something difficult because we might fail. Our ego would like life to be painless and blissful all the time and gets disappointed any time it is not. We need to stay alert and notice when our ego wants to discourage us from trusting all together. Remember, the immature ego sees things in terms of all or nothing, good or bad, black or white. The ego only wants to trust when it gets what it wants.

The immature ego is like a child that cannot wait. But the soul is comfortable wearing the trusting face of Eve and knows that life will bring what we need to grow. We gain self-knowledge, self-acceptance and self-love as long as we are open and willing to grow.

Great wisdom comes with this the veiled face of Eve. Eve ate the forbidden apple because she wanted knowledge above all. She trusted the urge to increase her awareness of reality. Her act was not one of mere rebellion and pride; she gave up the contentment of paradise in order to become more like God herself through the path of self-knowledge.

From this perspective, the serpent that tempted Eve may very well have been the Kundalini energy coming up from her root chakra and compelling her to become aware of her sexual energy. At the urging of the serpent, she left behind the shallow life of contentment to experiment with choice. For through choice, we create and become more God-like. Yes, Eve, and those of us who dare to wear her hidden faces, must deal with the contrast between good and evil, but she and we are also becoming a creator, not just a creation. Eve trusted the call to become a responsible creator.

120

## Lesson: Trust Who You Dance With

Tango, like any relationship, requires trust that you can stay on your own axis and that if you loose it your partner will help. Trust your choice. Continue to deepen your self-knowledge by finding out more about yourself in the dance of relationship. It takes two to Tango.

## Exercise for the Woman:

Go to a Milonga and look around to spot someone who might be compatible to dance with. You can see and feel if the man is dancing to show off his steps or dances to create joyful connection with the woman. When he invites you to dance say "yes" and feel your deep breathing relaxing your face, shoulders and legs. You connect with the muscles of the belly and the muscles in the back of your ribcage to ask them to hold your center strong with at the same time softening the front of your heart. Imagine that you your spine is kept erect by a spiral of light that lifts you to the sky while your limbs are loose and free.

Imagine that your central spiral is always spiraling in front of him connecting with your breath and your intention to open your heart to his way of hearing and following music. Start feeling your feet pressing against the floor and your head rising. Complete the embrace by holding your right hand with his left hand and your rests on his left arm. Pay attention to the shifts of weight that he's making to find out where your weight is before he starts moving.

This is the beginning of the dance. It starts with taking the time to establish trust.

## Exercise for the Man:

Go to a Milonga and watch how women are dancing. Are they waiting for the initiation of the next step by the man? Or are they rushing to the next step by themselves and the man feels pulled by her?

Are they holding their own balance while they energetically *enter* the man's chest melting with him and even feel from his breath how the softness or the power that he will put in the next step?

How well can she be fully relaxed in her chest and at the same time free in her hips so that round movements can engender a dance that is smooth and sensual? How loose are her legs while she's following his heart?

Then you might want to choose a woman that has all those qualities developed and enjoy the dance. Or if you feel generous, you might at times enjoy the challenge of dancing with someone who is just beginning paying special attention to your lead so she can follow more easily and feel encouraged.

# 9 Dynamic Balance

Of all the hidden faces of Eve, balance is one of the most challenging for women to grow into and wear with ease. The constant engagement with her inner masculine in pursuit of balance can reap great rewards, and the same is true of a man who deeply engages his inner feminine. A truly balanced individual possesses a deep inner calm that cannot be thrown off by anything that happens in the outer world.

This type of calm is not the result of avoiding feelings or conflicts. This is the calm that comes out of a deep recognition that you are connected with the entire cosmos and therefore can access whatever is needed to deal with life's many twists and turns. This type of calm makes it nearly impossible for the world to knock you off-center. This is the calm that sends roots down through your feet reaching deep into the belly of mother earth.

The challenge this face of Eve presents a woman is to fully embrace and develop her masculine aspect as a balanced complement to her femininity. We have Carl Jung to thank for deepening our understanding of the masculine and feminine traits or aspects that exist within each gender. Jung named the feminine soul expression of a male *anima* and the male soul expression of a female *animus*.

That both masculine and feminine traits exist in each gender is now commonly understood. Both men and women have the capacity to express the full spectrum of human traits. In many ways what is considered masculine versus feminine is culturally defined. What is more important to our discussion here is that both men and women long to merge and experience completion. We often look outside for that completion. A lack of balance inwardly can lead to troubled relationship dynamics. The more each person—man or woman—claims for him or herself the recessive traits they look to another to provide, the more successful the relationship with the other will be.

Eva Pierrakos explained this quite concisely in one of the Pathwork lectures when she said: The masculine principle expresses the outgoing movement of reaching, giving, acting, initiating, asserting. The feminine principle expresses the receptive movement: taking in, nurturing. In distortion and negativity, the masculine principle manifests as hostile aggression, hitting rather than giving and reaching. The feminine principle in distortion turns from loving receptivity and nurturing to grasping, grabbing,

*"Both men and women long to merge
and experience completion"*

stealing, holding tight, catching, and taking and not letting go.

The challenge for both sexes is to integrate the qualities of the opposite gender without losing or diminishing the traits of his or her gender. This integration, or at the very least a conscious awareness and willingness to work with the challenge it presents, opens the door to healthy relating. Of course, on the way to finding balance we often overshoot the mark. Often, as a woman embraces her animus, she will lose or diminish her femininity. Likewise, a man can get in touch with his feminine side and lose contact with his masculine core or favor the feminine side of his nature for any number of reasons.

On the beautiful island of Maui, this gender tension plays itself out in some curious ways. Maui is an exquisitely feminine place. Hula, the island goddess of dance, is all embracing; her nurturing energy gracefully touches everyone who visits the island. She delights in dancing with the heart of all her children and visitors. The island of Maui is quite literally enchanting, so much so that it is often referred to with the feminine pronoun *she*. Here, the oceans are warm and deeply blue. Maui winds have a quality of graceful dance like nowhere else. Her vegetation is luxurious, varied, and sensuous.

But an odd pitfall befalls some men who come to live in this paradise if they are not keen in their own pursuit of balance. The combination of such a feminine environment and the laid-back lifestyle on Maui lays the trap of this pitfall. Certainly, this situation is not isolated to Maui. The tendency among new age men to be

*"On the way to finding balance
we often overshoot the mark"*

"too soft" in the name of being spiritual is the subject of many a frustrated women's circle.

From the masculine perspective, this gender confusion is compounded by women's complaints about *macho men*. But the confusion can readily be cleared up if we make a distinction between *macho* and *strong*. A macho man feels superior to the woman and often uses his strength inappropriately to dominate her. A strong man is a balanced man.

*The sexual force is an expression of consciousness reaching for fusion and both masculine and feminine energy are needed to co-create this fusion.* Sometimes the female takes the initiative and sometimes the man does or the two can switch roles escalating pleasure until they reach the full fusion of orgasm. Neither men nor women need stay rigid in their primary gender role.

Many roles in life require a necessary switching between the masculine and feminine aspect. For instance, a mother is often in her masculine role when she feeds, instructs, and directs her children, then switches into a feminine role when she receives the pleasure of their smiles and giggles.

In both men and women, the feminine aspect can be out of balance and manifest as extreme passivity as if he or she were a piece of wood floating along in a river. Passively waiting for something to happen with no inner movement at all is a typical imbalanced feminine expression. The missing element is the inner movement: tuning in and evaluating what the flow brings in the way of opportunity, coincidence, and invitation toward outer

128

The balanced feminine doesn't simply wait—

she waits to see what looks most delicious.

Then, she is quick and savvy in how she activates

her masculine to take action.

movement. The balanced feminine doesn't simply wait—she waits to see what looks most delicious. Then, she is quick and savvy in how she activates her masculine to take action. While the feminine does not want to miss the newness that life has to offer, the masculine tracks prior commitments and obligations that could interfere with the new experience.

The balanced person whose masculine and feminine sides are in harmony will take responsibility for the entire situation and communicate accordingly.

The balanced female always has an instant connection with her masculine aspect. She is not afraid to take decisive action. Likewise, the balanced masculine always has his finger on the pulse of his feminine side. He is not out of touch with nor afraid of his emotions. For both genders, creating a fluid connection between these two vital aspects of the whole and complete self brings greater joy and fulfillment. Achieving this fluidity takes work and patience, however, as it involves maturing our immature aspects.

When we get lost in an immature, reactive emotional or mental pattern, several steps can be taken to find our way back to balance. The first and most powerful step we can take is to *become aware*. Simply noticing when either your feminine or masculine aspect is expressing from an immature or out-of-balance place will break the trance of that state of mind.

By state of mind I mean both thinking and feeling; the two are often fused in neural pathways and circuits that feel nearly impossible to re-route once they get activated. This is critical to

130

understand if we are to gain some perspective and objectivity. Humans are remarkably vulnerable creatures, especially when it comes to the contents of our subconscious mind. The patterns of imbalance can readily sweep us up; this is commonly called *getting triggered* or *being in reaction*. In order to break the pattern, defuse the trigger and unravel the reaction, we must *decide* to connect with the mature part of us. The mature feminine and the mature masculine can be well developed in our consciousness but they recede in the face of reactivity.

Choosing to connect with that mature aspect allows this more developed side to come forward and *respond* rather than react to a stimulus. This does not always happen as quickly as we'd like but once the storm of reaction has passed we can find a balanced perspective again. From this place of clear seeing, all the wisdom attained by the collective is available to us. This is the practical meaning of *we are all one.* The person who is truly humble enough to ask can access the wisdom of the ancients and all the great masters, including living masters. Only by choice can we clear the interference of mind and old patterns so we can listen to the wisdom within. This is the purpose and intent of meditation. And lastly, we decide to implement that wisdom.

This sequence—notice, decide to connect, re-establish balance, get quiet enough to clear out static from old beliefs, and decide to implement the wise choice—works every time. When emotions are strong, we may find it hard to slow down enough to go through the steps but we can always come back later and still reap the benefits.

This happened not long ago when I had a difficult confrontation with a friend over the beautiful Balinese floor tiles on my lanai in Maui. I was told I had a surplus of tiles and, neglecting to do the math myself, lent a number of boxes to a friend. Later, when I discovered that I had in fact come up short, I alerted my friend and asked him to make good on his promise to replace the tiles. I'd been waiting for the replacement tiles a full year when a crew of workers was out at the temple laying the last section of the floor. It was clear they would run out of tiles by mid-day. I made several phone calls that morning to track down my friend, asserting my need for the tiles right away. At some point, not having received any answer, I got in my car and drove toward his house to see if perhaps he was out of earshot from the phone. We met on the dusty road that leads to his house. He stopped his car and yelled out, "I have some boxes in the trunk of the car."

When I asked him to drive them over to my house one mile away to unload them for me, his facial expression became distorted with anger. He seemed possessed as he got out of his car, opened the trunk, picked up the boxes of tiles, and threw them on the dirt road. Without a word, he sped off in his car. I stood there, stunned, looking at the torn boxes lying on the dirt road. My energy completely froze.

Confused and hurt, my mind kept asking: *Why did he do that?* Fear activated a defensive pattern that locked me into a mental process. This type of mind-spin cuts me off from my heart and feelings; unfolding events can no longer be seen for what they are

132

and dealt with successfully. This type of mind-spin is one of many ways by which we *manage* intense emotions. Stranded in the mind, we try to grasp the *why* of the situation and avoid feeling the intensity of the confusion and hurt the situation stirred up. In the moment, it is easier to think through a difficult and painful situation than to feel it fully, especially when rejection is involved.

In this instance, I was caught up in that mental exercise for the better part of a day. I was trapped in a vicious circle. To break the vicious circle, I sat and chanted the heart chakra chant until I became more balanced. Finally, I became more interested in finding my center than being *right* about my friend having acted like a jerk. Aware that I had been in a reactive pattern, I went through the aforementioned sequence. By really listening to *his perspective* on what had happened that afternoon the way to restore balance with my friend opened up.

Reactive patterns are often quite blinding; they challenge us to open our seeing and balance our version of what has occurred with another person's point of view.

A problem with the tile manufacturer in Bali had made it impossible for my friend to replace the tiles in a timely fashion despite his efforts. Expecting at the very least a *"thank you,"* he was angered when I *demanded* that he bring the tiles over to my property and unload them for me. Apparently my demand shot out of me with a distorted, unbalanced masculine energy that he registered as overt hostility. This triggered a matching dynamic in him. We both lost our balance and could not connect with our mature selves.

Thankfully, after a while we both saw the humor in the whole situation. I felt humbled by the experience and realized that in a difficult situation I am not always immediately able to switch to the mature side of me. Yet, as they say: *better late than never.*

When we are in balance we are flexible with going into either our feminine or masculine or both depending on what is required in the moment. This allows us to avoid making a mess that we have to clean up later. Had I been able to stay in balance I would have gracefully thanked my friend for taking the time to bring the tiles to my place. I would have asked him to help me transfer the boxes into my car to save him the trip up Hana Highway to my property.

*For those of us who live life as an adventure, balance can be misinterpreted as boring. However, my experience of Tantra has revealed that quite the opposite is true. Staying in a balanced state of being can be quite thrilling.*

It requires special skills—just like any other high adventure activity.

Practicing Tantra allows us to develop this skill, a subtle but distinct inner movement to connect with all the energy centers so that we speak or act from the center of our being. Every moment can become an invitation to subtly reorient to the depths of our mature heart rather than the reflex of our *persona*. On the other hand, even the juiciest dramas become predictable when repeated over and over again. These are the *stuck places* that have the potential to bring the hurts we have not yet come to terms with and healed to the surface.

For instance, Jack came to me complaining that he no longer could make love to his wife Sonia with the passion he had felt early in their relationship. Four years earlier, Jack had fallen in love with Sonia. Her extreme emotionality was one of the traits that attracted him the most. Being a lawyer, he tended to be very rational and Sonia's freedom of expression exhilarated him.

As we know, opposites attract but the work of smoothing the edges of opposite traits remains to be done if a good relationship is what we want. Most couples do not see this need at first and fly through the *in love* phase then one day wake up hating the very quality they once loved in their partner.

At the beginning of their relationship, Sonia's emotions stimulated Jack and he greatly enjoyed her intensity. When she got angry over an occurrence at her job, a disagreement with a girlfriend, or simply having misplaced a blouse, he remained relaxed and calm. In the face of her regular fits of rage, which included beating her fists into the couch, he would feel amused. Sonia would say, "I hate this. I don't want to live anymore if life is so stinky," and Jack would sit back and enjoy the show. Inwardly, he would tell himself: *she is not serious about killing herself… this is really just a small upset; she is more intelligent than that… gosh, she's cute when she's mad!*

But Jack had grown tired of this behavior and no longer enjoyed the show. Sonia's complaining and acting out had become a consistent habit that tainted their daily lives with frustration. He wanted to come home to a peaceful place. Sonia's immature parts drove her to exaggerate even the smallest inconveniences into major catastrophes. Her dramas had become predictable and Jack was bored.

When the balanced feminine and the balanced masculine meet they find creative ways of responding to whatever life presents. As the interest in getting to know each other more deeply increases so does the sexual spark.

The centaur, a symbol of Sagittarius, is an excellent representation of what I perceive as essential in a mature, balanced human. We rise up out of our animal nature but are not separate from our instinctual self. Our body has all the needs and survival instincts of an animal. We need to eat, drink, sleep, and rest just like other animals. We are also human, however, and have a need to know, to be creative, to be autonomous and yet also connected with others. Our higher human needs call us to be artistic, to make a difference, to express ourselves romantically and poetically, to become aware of the duality that we live in and integrate it.

Let's consider one of the many pairs of needs—the need for autonomy and the need for connection. It is tempting to think these needs are antithetical. We can either be autonomous or connected but not both. In some couples, one person handles the connectivity while the other takes charge of ensuring autonomy. While these two human needs look contradictory only on the surface, in reality, they are simultaneous. Deep connection cannot happen if we do not also have the option to be autonomous when appropriate. The extreme example of this is what we call co-dependence.

*"The wholeness that we come from*
*and long to return to nudges us gently*
*to integrate the dualities of this physical life"*

The wholeness that we come from and long to return to nudges us gently to integrate the dualities of this physical life. If the gentle nudges don't move us toward becoming more whole then life may serve up a more startling jolt. The hidden face of Eve knows to take action and request the help of spirit. When we sincerely request help from our spirit, help always comes. The connection with spirit is always available and helps us calm the mind by opening the door to the heart where we *simply know*. This simple knowing in the spiritual heart makes it easy to integrate not only the more obvious dualities like black and white, or good and evil, but also the more subtle and challenging ones, like body and spirit, or sex and love.

The body is made of divine substance just as are the mind and emotions. The *essential stuff*, as Deepak Chopra calls it, expresses as body, mind, and spirit—each at a unique vibration or frequency. We could say that the body is slower moving spirit, more than simply a temple of the spirit, an expression of spirit in the flesh. Although a dense manifestation of the essential stuff, the body can be raised in its vibrational level through intentional practices such as are taught in the many branches and systems of yoga. Tantra teaches us to raise the vibrations of each energy center and spiral the alchemically modified energy of the lower centers into the higher centers until the body is literally made lighter.

In both Tantra and Tango a continuous stream of breath between the partners keeps the energy moving. Initially, this breath stream is intentional; it becomes automatic as waves of breath begin to flow between two bodies without effort. Tremendous pleasure comes with this merging on the wave of shared breath.

Balancing our lives can be accomplished by moving back and forth between different realities: the physical reality experienced by the spirit enjoying the body and the spiritual reality wherein we vibrate faster than our bodies. In this space we identify with the spirit/soul and the body becomes a temple of the spirit. Our soul is already one with all that exists. Then the soul comes back into the body and enjoys the five senses fully including the sixth sense of intuition. The senses become a means to take us deeper into our soul. This weaving back and forth between realities helps reaffirm the trust that we have acquired—many times and then forgotten—that we are all one. The more often we shift realities consciously the sooner we enter the state of complete peace and balance.

Balance is essential if we are to unmask all the hidden faces of Eve and fully flower as women. The same is true for the man who longs for personal mastery. Only in a balanced state can we really experience the One true reality. This was Eve's great leap in consciousness: to become aware and awake in a larger reality she had to risk eating that forbidden apple.

Some people are so in love with each other when they first meet that they don't have to think how to make each other happy and deepen the relationship. It seems to happen as of by itself with no effort at all. As a matter of fact you can't wait to spend quality time with each other and talk a lot. You do so much eye gazing naturally that when you go to a restaurant to eat you forget to order food until you are reminded.

Tantra tells us and experience proves that unfortunately after the first period of falling in love is over (usually between 6 months and 2 years) the newness that created that high seems to have fallen into habits. You think you know everything about your lover and start paying less attention to each other.

Now we enter into the phase of the relationship when it requires work to keep it fresh and alive and, unfortunately, most of us prefer to think that we are so connected that we can concentrate on our career instead.

This is the first mistake. Let's look at an analogy: how would it be if you got into a business partnership with someone that you like and trust and then you stop paying attention to the enterprise that you had started together? How successful would you imagine the business would be? Liking your partner is not going to make the business flourish unless you actually work together.

Logic tells us that if we don't keep working on our love partnership then we are not going to succeed. We need to focus on keeping our fire burning and Tantra teaches us how to do it. Here are some of the things that we need to continue paying attention to for the love relationship to continue to blossom and deepen.

## Lesson: Making Time for Love

We all know that love is most important in our life. At the moment of death everyone wishes that he/she had loved more. The more we

140

will have loved the less afraid of death we will be. Loving is living life fully. Only people who have not loved fully are afraid of dying because they have not lived fully.

Make love your priority. Making time for your beloved is a real statement of love.

**Exercise:**

Schedule days on your calendar to remind you which one of these suggestions you want to pay special attention to on that day.

- Plan a time that you can set aside to consciously make love spontaneously and pay attention to the newness of the moment every time you connect. Habits tend to numb love so try not to do the exact same thing that you always do.

- During the day take time to connect with your own erotic energy by taking deep slow breaths often, at least every two hours.

- When you meet with your lover look into his or her eyes to express your desire, your admiration, and your tenderness. The eyes can express all of it. Imagine how your eyes light up when you see a beautiful baby, a kitten, or a puppy, that is a tenderness look. Imagine how your look changes when you see a sexy scene. That is a desire look, and so on. Practice looking at each other with different expressions.

- Synchronize your breath with each other (breathing in and breathing out at the same time; if one of you is breathing faster than the other, slow down to match the slower of your two breaths). Do this for at least 2 minutes. You might discover that you suddenly *just know* what your lover is feeling.

- Notice and express what is right about each other. Become a finder of what you love in the other person. Most couples, once the initial falling in love phase has passed, become accustomed to paying attention to what needs to be corrected in their partner instead.

- When something is not working, tell your lover about it in a compassionate way, expressing your needs and desires as a gentle request instead of as a demand. If you are scared to express yourself because of previous conditioning, tell them as soon as possible that you are anxious and afraid to ask for what you want but that you are going to risk it anyway because you want to be connected and share all of you. The deeper that you go into truth the higher you go into ecstasy. Holding back from expressing your deep needs (and hoping that your partner guesses them) creates separation.

- Create a space in your home that is dedicated to love-making decorated in a way that takes you into an exotic space beyond the habitual.

  When you come home make a conscious choice to leave your survival worries at the door and enter your home as a temple of connection and love. After connecting in love then you can bring up your problems if you have any. Tantra suggests that rather than offering solutions just listen to your lover with compassion and full attention. Often this is all our lovers need to regain the strength to take care of it themselves. Unless you are specifically asked, "Would you please help me with this?" don't offer advice, especially if you are a man.

- Surprise each other with something that makes your heart sing. Even a simple call from the office to talk about what you imagine your lovemaking in the evening will be like starts the juices flowing.

  When you touch each other feel the love from your heart entering your partner's body even before your hand reaches theirs. Stay connected with your breathing so you always know where your lover is energetically and emotionally. This will help you know how to change your touch as you continue. If you are uncertain, gently ask your lover how he or she would like to be touched in that moment.

- Pay attention to your lover and you will have a rich source of real compliments to offer. Simply noticing lets your lover know he or she is important to you. Just to say, "I love you" or "you are beautiful" is not quite as powerful as letting your lover know how you feel and how much you care. For example, notice with precision something about your lover. Here are some instances of specific ways of saying "I love you":

  1) "When I look into your eyes I can see your devotion and I want to make love to you,"

2) "This morning you were wearing your beautiful red dress that brings out who you are, and I've been thinking of you all day,"

3) "When I listened to the genuine conversation you had this morning with our son I felt so happy that I married such a good father,"

4) "I can really notice how your muscles are getting stronger. Thank you for caring so much about your body."

Remember that a woman wants to be noticed and fully seen on all levels. A man wants to be acknowledged for his manly body and his contribution to your life. Usually he receives enough strokes for his mind and accomplishments and not enough for his body.

*"The deeper that you go into truth the higher you go into ecstasy.*
*Holding back from expressing your deep needs*
*creates separation"*

# 10 Creativity and Self-Actualization

During a recent outing to Ho'okipah Beach on the east side of Maui, I had the great pleasure of watching a baby playing in the sand and practically jumping out of her skin with joy. With her hands and whole body, she cheered the ocean waves as they splashed onto shore. The sounds that flowed out of her in a wave of little-girl-glee may have been incomprehensible in terms of syntax, but every adult within earshot understood her bubbling joy.

Then, sitting in the sand, the little one pedaled with her feet and pushed the sand into a pile. She giggled, happy to have made such a high wall of sand and smiled at her mom with great satisfaction. The next moment she exploded into a frenzy of movement with her hands scattering the wall of sand. Clapping her wet, sandy hands, she giggled and screamed while a thrill of great pleasure spread her joy to all who witnessed her creative burst of energy.

In babies, creativity expresses itself spontaneously. They have an impulse and execute it right away. No long plans, no inner conflict—they just do it. Creativity is an instinct we all have that serves our survival. Creativity is a very essential quality. We all are born creative. Depending on both life circumstances and on the character of the individual, we either develop our creativity or stifle it out of fear that we might make a mistake and/or encounter disapproval.

When I was a child my parents had no money to buy toys but to my eyes anything in sight was a potential toy. A smooth peace of wood became a doll. A small rake became a tool to make deep lines on the earth that resembled streets. Little stones of different shapes placed along those imaginary streets and, voila! I had created a village complete with houses, stores, and school.

Around age four or five I found a beautiful old carved chest hidden behind a pile of wood. My imagination started to go wild. Perhaps it had belonged to a queen! I opened it carefully and to my amazement found a pile of colorful shawls and rich fabrics. These were surely the elegant accessories of a queen. How would it feel to wear a royal garment? As I pulled out an especially decorative shawl and draped it around my shoulders an unexpected transformation happened as if by magic. My body seemed to grow taller and fuller. Servants appeared, ready to fulfill my every wish. I walked through a grand room filled with gorgeous works of art and ornate furniture then passed through a set of ornate French doors into a beautifully groomed garden. As I began to parade around, the trees and shrubs changed into my subjects and bowed. I greeted them each with a soft smile waving to all of my subjects with open hands and an open heart. I joyously spread love and blessings to my people.

*Through creative imagination I discovered that I could be kind and loving while holding a powerful position.*

This moment of imaginary *Queenhood* canceled my fears that I might hurt people if given power. That's what I'd been told: "powerful people do bad things." Healing can happen through imagination.

Another afternoon, mother and I were raking the hay when the sun started to sink into the horizon. I was eight years old at the time and mother told me to go home and cook up something for supper.

"What should I cook?" I asked.

"Potatoes," she replied.

Never having cooked potatoes before, I asked how long they should cook. Mother answered, annoyed: "You'll find out."

Scared to ask her to be more specific, I decided to guess. After the potatoes had been boiling ten minutes I poked them with a fork. They were still hard so I tested them again and again. By the time the potatoes finally became soft enough to eat they had so many holes that they looked like a colander used to drain pasta. Knowing I was in for a stiff dose of ridicule from my family over this faux pas, I got busy. First, I carved little holes in the potatoes to disguise the pokes and then brushed them with butter and filled in the holes

*"Healing can happen through imagination"*

with grated cheese. Not only did the dish l

fantastic.

Like many a new innovation, this little bit (

came out of a feeling of desperation which in my

being ridiculed. The result not only brought me j‍          ‍‍‍u my

fragile self-esteem it gave me clear evidence that I could come up

with a brilliant solution when I found myself in a fix.

As a student I was gifted with another kind of creativity. When

we behaved especially well in school our teacher would read us

stories as a reward. I loved to hear my favorite teacher read those

stories and would listen closely all the while creating pictures in my

mind. I had a knack for going beyond the words into highly

symbolic realms. The symbols were always clear to me. When the

teacher would explain the symbolism to the class her description

matched almost perfectly what I had imagined. This kind of

creativity has helped throughout my life and allows me to

understand people and situations on many different levels.

As a Passionate Relationship guide and Tantric Healer, this type

of creativity also helps me to understand my clients on many levels

by enabling me to see and hear what they may not be willing or able

to verbalize. This, in turn, allows me to ask questions that reveal

levels they may not even realize that they are trying to hide. I then

encourage acceptance and compassion and help them to embrace

hidden—and quite often rejected—parts of themselves. A few of

my clients called my approach laser-beam psychotherapy.

The creative impulse kicked in big time when I gave birth to my son. I was nearing the end of my pregnancy and living alone after having separated from my husband over a secret affair he had been conducting with a friend of mine while I was carrying our child. Having made a decision to raise the child alone rather than put up with his infidelities, I was very sad about my situation and nervous about going into labor. I was not looking forward to delivering the baby alone and impatiently awaited the start of the contractions.

I was living in Berlin at the time, and the time for Mardi Gras had arrived. Germans love to dress up for Masquerade and dance all night and I was tired of sitting around waiting for the contractions to start. I thought: *if I go out dancing the contractions might come sooner perhaps helped by the movement.* With the speed of a young girl and the thoughtfulness of a grown-up I prepared the bag I would need at the hospital, put on a touch of make up, found something sexy to disguise my big belly, and a put on a mask of Cleopatra. The costume worked; no one guessed I was about to give birth. I was a voluptuous Cleopatra rather than a pregnant woman. I tucked the phone number for a taxi inside my bra just in case the contractions were to start and went off to the Masquerade.

After three hours of high energy dancing the contractions started coming. I asked the young man I was dancing with to call a taxi saying, "I have to get to the hospital, I'm about to give birth!"

My son was born after little more than two hours labor.

The most difficult moments of our lives often elicit surprising creativity. The pressure cooker of a no-win situation can pop the lid

*"The most difficult moments of our lives often elicit surprising creativity"*

ıght we were. Entirely new ways of being and new

expand our sense of what we can and cannot do.

Eve is discovered at pivotal moments in our lives but

in no-pressure situations once we know it's there. Engaging this side of ourselves on a regular basis strengthens and grows our creativity. Resolving conflicts can provide us with such strengthening practice.

As author Ronald Heifetz (*Leadership Without Easy Answers*, 2002, Harvard Business School Press) said, "Conflict is the primary engine of creativity and innovation. People don't learn by staring into a mirror; people learn by encountering difference."

A life well-lived involves creativity on all levels. Even love is an expression of creativity from the part of us that wants to embrace another to create a larger ONE. When creative juices flow we feel light, inspired, and happy. The part of us that is habituated fights this urge—all it wants to do is rest and enjoy what already is. "Why this constant drive to give of yourself?" the habitual self asks.

Can you tell a tree to hold back its fruits? The difference between a tree and you or me is that a tree does not experience inner conflict about growing its fruits. Neither does a tree judge its fruits as good or bad. The tree simply allows creation to happen. In a sense, the tree has no choice, just as Eve had no choice *before* she ate the fruit. Yet Eve wanted choice and the consequence of her action included feeling the tension of duality pulling her in two directions.

When I left my village at the age of thirteen, two primary forces were at work. First, the pain of not feeling loved or understood seemed to be pushing me out the door. But another force was equally strong—the pull to discover what more was inside me. I knew this could not happen in my village.

The story of Galileo had struck a deep cord in me and I felt certain I was destined for the life of an outcast if I stayed. Galileo's creative nature had led him to many remarkable discoveries, and yet he was imprisoned when he would not retract his theory that the Earth was not the center of the Universe. He was treated like a criminal when he refused to comply with the *authorities* and disprove his own scientific proofs that the Earth was, in fact, round. The church tribunal refused to look at those proofs and charged Galileo with heresy.

This story put quite a spin on my budding adolescent view of the world. I will not end up like Galileo, I thought to myself. I did not feel I would discover something scientific but I would discover something about men and women and God and I was sure I could not do so in my village. If Galileo—with all the strength of solid science behind him—had been rejected for his pioneering ideas then my chances of discovering different ideas about those subjects in a narrow-minded village were pretty slim. I hoped the larger world would be more likely to embrace my creative imagination. I imagined my distant future as a teacher in a place that was more open-minded.

*Looking back I can clearly see that a large part of my creativity has always revolved around the search for self-knowledge and my observations brought me to answers that could not be proven, only felt.*

My father had taught me well to trust my intuition. Some of his wildest imaginings eventually revealed themselves as not so wild after all. One day while we walked together through the woods he stopped to smell the pine needles. He put one in his mouth and started chewing. After a moment of deep reflection he said with conviction, "I think in the future people will eat the juice from pine tree and they will live longer." Many years later, while reading about the latest advances in nutrition, I learned that Pycnogenol comes from pine bark and has been confirmed to have powerful antioxidant properties that slow down the aging process. My father's creativity allowed him to see into the future.

While my father chose to dream and leave it at that, I longed to bring my dreams into reality. *A vision of creating a place to live where I would be surrounded by natural beauty remained in my mind and heart.* I could see this place in my mind's eye; it had a view of both a mountain and the ocean. This place would feel as nourishing as a good womb. Made of natural materials, it would feature different kinds of wood and marble and have a large outdoor bathtub surrounded by trees to afford privacy and yet be in nature. This place would remind me of my soul and have statues of Human Divinities who embody the qualities I want to nurture in myself. It would have to have a skylight and lots of windows to allow the feeling of being connected to the expanse of nature. From my dream place I would be able to see the sunrise and feel the magic it brings to every single day.

Today, on the enchanted island of Maui, I realized that vision by creating my temple/villa in Huelo on the way to exquisitely beautiful and romantic Hana coast. It is as though my inner female had dreamed up the villa and my inner male worked hard to make it happen. The villa is a visible co-creation of my inner male and female, who attracted the circumstances that actualized my goal. Its very existence has proved what I had always believed in my heart: that dreams can come true if we keep them alive and take the needed steps.

People who are bored with life do well to allow themselves to get in touch with their creative genius. Creativity is the face of Eve that expresses the higher potential she saw when she chose to eat the forbidden fruit: to be a conscious creator. To lift the veil that hides creativity can be challenging but absolutely rewarding.

Dance is one of the many ways to engage creativity. This joyous pastime can help you create a tangible connection with the Divine Feminine. This essential archetype loves to express—through both women and men—in all forms of dance; she uses the music to give rhythm to her infinite sound. At the end of the day I often drop in a CD of my favorite music and—depending on my mood—put on either a belly dance or Argentine Tango outfit. As the sound fills the room and my body, I allow the movement to come from within, letting go of steps learned. I surrender to the rhythm and have an exhilarating experience of unity: the music and I become one. Music can be a wonderful lover if allowed to enter you fully.

## Lesson: Moving with the Rhythm of Life

This practice is designed to help you re-discover that true self who wants to move to music. In truth we are all dancers because the spirit that moves in our body is dancing any time we take a breath.

*Life is movement.*

"But, I'm not a dancer!" you might say. Many people—both women and men—say this when I recommend movement to music. Somewhere along the line these men and women were likely to have been told that they had two left feet or heard some other derogatory comment from someone whose opinion mattered to them. Sometimes, people think they are doing you a favor by discouraging you from doing what you might feel embarrassed about instead of encouraging you to do your best.

Any negative remark could be enough to discourage you to dance your dance, whether to music or through life. You might want to invest time in discovering what beliefs you could change to be more fully expressive in your life. As a dance teacher I once had used to say: "You don't stop moving because you get old, you get old because you stop moving."

*Death is stagnation and decay.* Dance opens people up to move more energy. You can dance a very sexy dance moving your hips freely in different rhythms whether standing or lying down. You will

*"In truth we are all dancers because*
*the spirit that moves in our body is dancing*
*any time we take a breath"*

be surprised how much more pleasure you can feel dancing horizontally with your lover once you get comfortable and let yourself dance!

Dancing does miracles for self-esteem when practiced for the sake of self-love and creative expression.

## Exercise:

- Set aside a minimum of fifteen minutes for this exercise.
- Choose a favorite CD and clear an area at the center of a room.
- Start by lying on the floor and simply letting the music wash over you. Don't begin to move until you feel the music begin to move you.
- Let go of any notion about correct dance steps; your task is simply to discover how your insides want to move. Any judgment stifles your creativity and adds to poor self-image.

### Lesson: Eradicating deep beliefs that do not serve you

In exercise 1 and 2 below you will have an opportunity to unearth core beliefs that no longer serve you. Imagine you are digging a hole 20 feet deep (one foot for each affirmation of the new belief). As you dig into the soil of your subconscious, you will come upon obstructions—the rocks, weeds, old dead roots, and poisonous plants of contradictory beliefs that must be removed so that your new beliefs can take root and prosper. The digging process happens by repeating your chosen affirmation (the "new belief implant" that will support your growth and development) then taking a breath and

160

listening for thoughts that agree or disagree with the affirmation. After taking a deep breath, you will witness and let go of conflicting beliefs that might stifle the life affirming new belief. I will guide you through this process in the exercises below:

**Exercise 1:**

Take a sheet of paper and divide it in 2.

On the left side write your affirmation of the belief you want to implant 20 times at one sitting. It is important to keep digging down into the unconscious without interruption to achieve best results. For example: a man who was called a sissy as a young boy might have concluded that he is wimpy or some other discouraging belief.

He would start by writing on the left side of the paper: "I am an assertive and loving man." Each time he writes this phrase, he stops and checks the reaction in his body, imagining he has a special search light that can zero in on unconscious and subconscious contradictory messages deeply embedded in his mind.

On the right side of the page he writes down the thoughts he just discovered. After paying attention to cues his body might be giving him., such as such as tightening of some muscles, cringing, or headshaking as though to say "NO." His stomach could contract at the thought, "I am a wimp." Or "I'm scared that people won't like me."

Usually by the 15$^{th}$ repetition of the affirmation the negative responses calm down and you start to accept that you are in fact starting a new life guided by the new belief. In the case of our example—an assertive and loving man instead of a wimp.

I recommend you choose the affirmation you want to work with and do this exercise for 7 consecutive days.

**Exercise 2:**

If a sensitive girl constantly witnesses her mother yelling and screaming and in her pain decides, "I will not be like my mother," then the girl does not see healthier alternatives to screaming. She does not know that her mother could communicate what she wants clearly and harmoniously and be more likely to get what she wants. She might not even be able to conceive that her mother could communicate her needs and stay in conversation until she felt understood.

Take a sheet of paper and divide it in 2

Write the affirmation you are choosing to work with on the left side 20 times in one sitting. For example: "I am expressing my needs and I am heard." Each time you write your affirmation, stop and check the reaction of your body as discussed above.

On the right side of the page write down the contradictory thoughts as you did before.

Example: She notices that her throat starts contracting and detects the thought, "I am egotistical," or "I don't want to ask; it will break the peace that we have."

Usually by the 15th repetition of the new affirmation, the negative responses calm down and you start to accept that you are in fact starting your new life as an assertive and loving woman who has sacred needs. Needs are sacred because we are taking care of ourselves physically, emotionally and spiritually.

In addition to our needs for air, water, food, and rest, we have the need to love and to be loved, to be heard, to be seen, to connect with others, to express ourselves sexually, to have alone time, to contribute to life, and many more. There is a difference between being needy in a manipulative way and having needs that you have the right to fulfill if you want a satisfying life. A healthy family is happy to hear your needs. We all have the same basic needs but we don't always express them and when they are not fulfilled we get angry. The new contract expresses a healthier way of living a life that your spirit *enjoys* living.

I recommend you do this for 7 consecutive days. If the negative responses keep persisting you might need help from a professional to clear out the persistent negative thought and finally implant the new contract.

# 11 Make Love with the Divine

The more that we live and grow in self-awareness the more we realize that life is our greatest gift. The more we enter into and embrace the experience of duality, the more we see and understand that one aspect of reality cannot exist without the other. If we miss this realization in life we will surely grasp it at the moment of death according to many a near-death experience. The beauty of grasping the seamless whole of reality while we're alive cannot be understated. As the poet Kabir said:

> Friend, hope for the guest while you're alive.
> Jump into experience while you're alive.
> Think, and think while you are alive.
> What you call salvation belongs to the time before death.
> If you don't break your ropes while you're alive,
> do you think ghosts will do it after?
> The idea that the soul will join the ecstatic
> just because the body is rotten—

165

that is all fantasy.
What is found now is found then.
If you find nothing now,
you will simply end up with an apartment in the City of Death.
If you make love with the divine now,
in the next life you will have the face of satisfied desire.
So plunge into the truth, find out who the Teacher is,
believe in the Great Sound.

On their death-bed, no one has been known to say that they wish that they had never lived. On the contrary, many say they wish they had lived with more passion and loved more.

The many hidden faces of Eve (and I have only described a few) are comparable to the many facets of a diamond. The diamond of your true self is Pure Love. Just like a diamond in the raw, you may not reveal your brilliance until you have been refined and polished by life. Our true divine essence shines through when we do the inner work of uncovering the hidden brilliant faces. These faces, when revealed, are like mirrors reflecting divinity and bringing richness and depth to our lives. A great deal of careful work and attention goes into polishing a raw diamond, and rubbing against each other's visible faces helps us recognize the work we have to do. The yoga of relationship is a sure, although not necessarily easy, way to enlightenment.

Both Tantra and Tango require discipline and focus, and offer the pleasure of deep, loving connection along the way. We learn to dance through life consciously and to persist when the steps are not as smooth as we might like. Commitment to the path makes even clumsy moments full of beauty. The key is to keep coming back to an awareness of the now, to stay present and aware even in the difficult times. A mind that can stay focused is a meditative mind. Some people sit in meditation for hours at a time to achieve this depth of focus. I chose Tantra and Tango as my paths because my temperament is not inclined to sitting meditations. I like meditations in motion. And I am sure you can find the path that's for you, the dance that turns you on while you polish the divine diamond that you are.

I know how much intention and focus it takes to discover and experience just one of the faces of the divine. The good news is that the deeper you enter into a real understanding and integration of even one of those hidden faces, the easier it is to see and experience all the others. Once you reach into the deepest core of who you are, you will discover the faceless and nameless One: the essence of spirit, eternal God and Goddess, the vast dimension of pure being from which all faces and forms arise.

# Appendices

Appendix A

**Breathing**

There are two basic types of breaths, the Masculine or Shiva breath and the Feminine or Shakti breath.

There is little discussion on the Feminine Breath in tantric texts. Far more has been written about the Masculine Breath, which is more concerned with productive, goal oriented and disciplined practices. The feminine breath requires no effort on the inhalation, no holding of breath, and no controlled exhalation and it is completely natural.

Best described as Ocean Breath, this type of breathing is reminiscent of ocean waves that flow in a constant motion and do not stop at the crest to sustain their height. Next time you are near the ocean, notice how the waves behave, as soon as they reach the crest they fall onto the sand or rocks and then glide back into the ocean and a moment later, the next one is ready to come in. Waves come in cycles, each building on the last with increasing force until the highest wave is reached. Then the ocean sends smaller waves again and begins to build up to another big one in a constant, hypnotic movement. The size of the waves depends on the strength of the wind and the gravitation of the moon.

Throughout this book I refer to this style of Feminine Breathing alternatively as Ocean Breath, circular breathing, belly breathing, diaphragmatic breathing, open-mouth breathing depending on the context.

The Ocean Breath helps us:

- establish an almost immediate connection with our own Chakra system
- connect with the chakras of our lover
- bring to the surface emotions that might be stuck and difficult to express
- transmit heart energy through touch by synchronizing the transmission of love from the giver to the receiver during the exhalation and absorbing and integrating it during the inhalation
- increase oxygen intake
- relax the jaw and the throat
- create instant passage to the heart, the power, and the sex centers
- bypass the judgmental part of our mind so we can enjoy and stay in deep heart connection
- increase sensual awareness

I recommend initiating the tantric connection with the Ocean Breath because water is the element which corresponds to the sex center..

**The Masculine Breath** is a controlled breath. After the sensual and emotional energies have been stirred up and are vibrating in the body, we want to harness those energies in a purposeful way:

- to direct it to our higher chakras
- to direct it our lover's chakras to help them rise in love with us

- to transform sexual energy into higher spiritual energy and nourish the chakras by having multiple body orgasms without ejaculation.

The Cobra Breath can also be used for spiritual purification.

The Sanskrit word *pranayama*, refers to an entire science and study of breath control, which is a major component of every yoga system. Although most yoga books describe some form of pranayama, I recommend you learn directly from an experienced teacher. In this book I will limit my explanations to the synchronized breath used during soul gazing and the Cobra Breath.

To better understand the masculine, controlled breath, I recommend "The Science of Breath; A practical Guide" (*Swami Rama, copyright 1979 by the Himalayan International Institute in Pennsylvania*)

Appendix B

## Becoming Fully Potent

*Glossary of words used: lingam (penis), prana: life-force coming in especially through the breath, Yoni (vagina); Amrita, female ejaculate, "Goddess Nectar"*

Although we don't often think of impotence, whether due to physical or psychological causes, as a debilitating affliction However, impotence can be quite disturbing for a man. Confusion about how to deal with the condition causes a great deal of grief and disappointment. Men—and their partners—often report feeling "cheated" by life.

Impotence can occur at various levels from non-performance to inadequate performance and the causes can be physiological or psychological. To eliminate the possibility of a physiological cause I recommend you see a medical doctor or urologist for an evaluation.

If you are physically normal and still are faced with a recurring challenge and have difficulty getting and keeping a strong erection, rest assured and be encouraged because Tantra offers solutions to this common problem.

Possible causes of impotence are emotional or psycho-spiritual:
- an old guilt that was never addressed
- some fear of getting old
- a hidden shameful experience that suddenly reemerges during lovemaking, for example: someone criticized you as a lover or made fun of your lingam.

When we are young we have enough energy to suppress the damaging effects of shame, guilt, or abuse, and still manage to function adequately. As we get older the energy available to suppress negative events and emotional states lessens and the suppressed material starts coming up into consciousness and causing trouble. We can see this in older people who have not done their healing work—their defenses become calcified and they can appear like a caricature or a parody of themselves. Whereas people who did and continue doing their healing work have more energy available and are flexible in their character.

Other causes can include:

- stress at work
- fear of losing a job
- stress in the relationship with your love partner
- hidden anger that you do not clearly admit to feeling.

A common pattern I see among men is a tendency to avoid unpleasant communications, conditioned as they are by the often times explosive reactions of women. Unfortunately, avoidance leaves the angry feelings unaddressed and swept under the proverbial rug where they begin to fester. If a man does not have an outlet for these feelings—either a men's group or some other supportive relationship—they may create a block to intimacy and hot sex.

Tantra addresses these issues holistically and encourages the development of self-knowledge. Once you see through to your personal truth and learn loving and efficient ways to communicate and create the highest sexual flow, you will discover what many have: that *truth is a remarkable aphrodisiac.*

Sometimes worrying about impotence alone makes it worse. Over concern or anxiety about losing an erection or being unable to get physically aroused exacerbates the problem.

Tantric techniques can help you relax and enjoy being intimate whether or not you have an erection. Learning to relax is the first step. For most men, breaking free of the mind and it's constant "surveillance" in the form of a running commentary about how you are "performing" leads to a big surprise in the form of a strong erection that lasts.

Tantra encourages a man to shift his focus, taking his attention off himself and his worries about performance and instead look into his woman's eyes. By concentrating on her beauty or her expression or the way she moves or her response to the movement of energy between you, men learn to go deeper into intimacy and break the trance of the judgmental mind that tells them how hard they should be at any given moment of love making!

Tantra recommends training the ever-busy mind to stay focused on the breathing and/or on the above tantric intimacy deepening techniques.

This is what you can do to help yourself attain a higher degree of potency:

- Pay attention to your breathing. With awareness, follow the air all the way to the bottom of your diaphragm feeling your belly and lower back gently expanding. This has at least three important effects:

1. It creates more energy because the lower part of the lungs contain more air
2. When the belly expands down it creates increased circulation
3. More sensations in the genitals

- Softening your lips and the back part of your tongue helps to direct the breath lower into the lungs by directing the inhalation down instead of up toward the brain
- Exhaling, making soft and relaxing sounds as if gently sighing during the exhalation such as the "aah" sound. This will keep you centered in your heart instead of in the head of your lingam.

Making sounds increases energy flow and excitement. Notice how your body starts enjoying the added energy that comes from this self-hypnotic relaxation. All these practices help to create a positive loop toward higher relaxed excitement.

- Enjoying the sensation of pleasant fullness and pulsations throughout the whole body. Yes, finally relaxing, no job to be performed, no goal to reach, just connecting with your self and your present state of being.

This wonderful relaxation is setting the stage for high-level lovemaking. Why? When you are that relaxed you can bring your attention toward your lover and at the same time remain fully present in your whole body, including the genitals, not just in the head (desire). Your being fully present is the major cause of your lover's excitement. Techniques without presence can be mechanical.

Your whole body is a bigger container of energy than your lingam alone and so you can contain more of the high pleasure without having to control it. Control, even tantric control, requires a certain tension. This is the time to release tension. You can really be present on all levels to feel the pleasure of giving or receiving, whatever wants to happen first.

Sometimes a woman loves to initiate the caressing and enjoys giving to you. She might caress, massage, or kiss you. In that case, just be in the receiving mode. I'm aware that this is not as easy as it sounds because to just receive means to give up control of the situation. Remember to breathe.

Often, some part of the mind tells us that our partner should be able to read us and know what we want in the moment. We might be either embarrassed to ask or disappointed that they did not read us perfectly.

Many men seem to find it challenging to receive. It is perhaps because culturally most men are taught that they must be on the giving side. These men can learn the wonderful skills of being present to receive fully:

- This is your time to receive and take in fully. Your gift to the giver is the pleasure of being completely received.

- Don't direct energy to your mind when it tells you that you should reciprocate. Remind yourself that when you receive all the pleasure she's giving, you are going to give her much more after you are fully engorged.
- Allow yourself to be filled and express your pleasure as much as possible. Gratefulness increases pleasure for the giver and the receiver.
- Deepen your breathing. Feel the expansion throughout your torso, allow the breath to reach down toward the sacrum or even the anus.

The lower you can imagine your air goes the fuller your lungs are going to become thus providing your blood with an increased amount of oxygen and life force. Blood is going to flood all of your organs and your lingam as well.

If you are in the mood for giving first please do so with the same attention.

- Pay attention to your breathing and to hers as well.
- If her breathing is shallow invite her to feel your hand on her belly and feel it rising and falling.
- Connect your hands with her yoni and her heart by holding your right hand on her yoni and your left on her heart until you feel her breathing deepen.
- Relax your touch when you inhale and intentionally fill yourself up with prana.

- Add energy to your touch when you exhale. She will feel your potency through your intentional touch.
- If you touch her on her belly or chest make sure you coordinate with her breath.

This will bring you much deeper and closer to your lover than you can imagine!

Use visualization:

- We know for certain that energy follows the mind. In other words energy goes to the place in your body where your focus is. If you are not good at visualizing **imagine** that you can feel the prana streaming through the body feeding all your organs, especially flooding your lingam and creating a tower of energy.

After the inhalation is completed the exchange of oxygen and carbon dioxide takes place. The rest of the body longingly awaits the new supply of oxygen and prana. It is at this point—the point between inhale and exhale—that we have the power to mentally direct where most of this energy should go.

The aim of most aphrodisiacs and sexual enhancement supplements, including Viagra, is to increase circulation in the sex organs. With practice, you can use the power of concentration and focus to achieve the same result any time you want to.

Mechanical and safe ways to experience a powerful erection:

- Have your lover hold the base of your sexual organ creating a comfortably tight ring around your scrotum and lingam. This allows for the blood to be temporarily trapped into your sexual organs thus building up engorgement.
- Or use a *cock ring*, best with a release button for comfort and safety.

Pleasurable techniques that utilize a soft lingam:
- A technique called *churning butter* in the Kama Sutra by moving your hips in circles and keeping the lingam pressed against the pubic mound so the lingam absorbs the warmth of the yoni while becoming solid 'like a piece of butter.'
- Rolling the lingam on and around the clitoris and up and down the vaginal lips.
- Stuffing a soft lingam into the yoni and moving side to side at different angles instead of in and out.

Find your own playful ways. If something you try does not give you the expected result then playfully scratch it off as an experiment. Make sure you are not adding it to a list of *failures*. The heaviness of such a list is definitely counterproductive.

Some men have a hard time training their mind to stay focused on the tantric breathing. For these men there might be other way to make themselves feel potent and powerful. They love to be made love to by their woman without direct stimulation. Direct stimulation might be too confronting if they don't respond with an erection as fast as they wish and that might contribute to make things worse. However, if their woman seduces them indirectly, perhaps by sensuously undressing herself or touching herself seductively, or by saying some sexy words, this can work wonders to raise her man's self-esteem as a lover.

Consider what happened for Nancy and Peter:

Peter loves Nancy very deeply and would do anything to make her happy. His greatest pleasure is in taking her into as many orgasms as she wants until she's so full of pleasure that at almost every touch she has another orgasm, a wave of orgasms, just as the waves of the ocean constantly follow each other.

The challenge that Peter has is that he needs her to start the seduction so that he feels very wanted as a man. However, when his mind and heart get turned on he is unable to transfer that energy to his lingam and keep it present there long enough to have powerful intercourse.

His mind is attacked by thoughts of porno movies showing men with an 18 inch lingam shoving it relentlessly, and with full force, into the woman while muttering derogatory words, with an angry face. He would never use that kind of approach with his beloved Nancy. He cannot imagine himself using this kind of approach. So he holds back and becomes soft and *tender.*

It is very difficult for Nancy to get to very high sexual places with him because she likes to be seduced and *taken.* She would love for Peter to take the leading role in the love play and almost be taken by force.

The problem that this couple has is that what means love to her would mean abuse in Peter's mind. And he is too nice a man to abuse her.

Peter does not understand that once he takes her she would become very open to his loving and gentle approach and at this point he could give her all the tenderness that they both deeply want and desire.

When he takes on the role of powerful masculinity—as seen by Nancy—she would become the powerful feminine who would first surrender fully to the lovemaking he would initiate. After that, when full, she naturally would switch roles and become the tigress and active lover that he's dreaming of.

They both understand this. Nancy decides to take the initiative against her 'natural preference' and starts undressing sexily for him. This, to her surprise, starts to turn her on also and she gets more deeply into her seductive role.

Placing herself so that he has to look up to her, she started massaging her body with long sensual strokes that start at her inner thighs and continue through her already pulsating yoni and circling around her belly. She continues by massaging her breasts, encircling each breast with her two hands, lifting her breasts gently, and ending the sexy circles with a squeeze of her already erect nipples. She does this while opening her mouth and licking her lips, sending him ecstatic sexy looks with her big eyes.

Flames of passion streamed out of her eyes because at this point she was no longer acting. She actually was enjoying being the seductress.

She asked Peter to masturbate and he was more than willing to comply. The intensity of the *scene* was so great that he forgot about the tantric preference of orgasm without ejaculation and he allowed his semen to squirt out. His orgasm was more forceful and the ejaculate more abundant then usual.

She avidly rubbed his ejaculate on her belly commenting how excited she was to see him so sexually charged. She then lay down next to him, naturally now in her soft, feminine approach.

The gratefulness he felt for what he had just received gave him such a great shot of energy that he started to rub his now soft lingam on her yoni, already moist from the excitement of the new experience of seductress. She then *stuffed* the flaccid lingam into her yoni. Her heat increased as she enjoyed his pelvis pressing on her pubic bone. He moved his hips in small circles allowing his lingam to plop outside of her and rub against her labia. He was now giving back to her all of his newly stirred up passion through his eyes.

Waves of orgasmic energy were now moving throughout her whole body. His lingam slowly became erect and almost purple with blood. He wanted to penetrate her sacred space (yoni), but she did not let him inside just yet. That made him even hotter and he then imagined entering her moist yoni and absorbing all that sweet nectar in her sacred cave. He imagined that his erection was perfectly

184

stimulating her sacred spot (g-spot) and after only a few strokes he continued imagining that she washed his happy lingam with hot Amrita. He was very surprised how easy it had been.

He related to me that what helped him send sexual energy into Nancy was the imagination of penetrating her with his *big* lingam. He felt his lingam had become bigger than he had imagined by absorbing her powerful energy. He imagined that he penetrated her all the way to her heart.

They enjoyed a nurturing afterglow exchanging loving looks and tender caresses. The sexual energy they had just stirred up was transforming into fuller love and spiritual connection. They discussed their dreams and realized that they both were thinking of a home/temple of their own that was conducive to love-making. They realized that this was the concept known as *Sex Magic*.

Shortly after the after-glow pause, sexual energy started flowing abundantly between them again. When they reached the highest peak they did three *Cobra Breaths* to bring that rich energy up to the Third Eye where they both empowered their vision.

The deep love that they felt for each other seemed to have extracted the essence of his seeds and her amrita, essence that they pulled up through the spinal cord into the brain, to give power to the seed of consciousness they both held as a vision in their foreheads at same time. It worked! They manifested their dream house only six months later.

They have understood that tantric lovemaking is more about moving energy and charging it with a focused mind than about erections and ejaculations.

Appendix C

**Female Ejaculation**

Does a woman ejaculate? The answer is a definite yes. With proper stimulation of the G-spot women can ejaculate a fluid from ducts located around the urethra. It is located in the front wall of the vagina under the pubic bone. This is a spongy area about two inches or more inside the yoni (vagina) depending on the size of the yoni and the location of the clitoris. It is actually the South Pole of the clitoris when laying on one's back.

Female ejaculation has been documented in ancient China and India where the 'Goddess-spot' massage was a common tantric-sex technique. Tantric texts call the liquid produce *amrita,* or "sweet nectar." It is a protein-based fluid found to be chemically different from urine. It is believed to have great healing properties.

This knowledge is slowly coming to the awareness of non-tantric people like Dr. Mitchell Levine, a gynecologist/obstetrician at the Women Care Clinic on the east coast, who declares that women do ejaculate. He believes that the hush-hush aura around the subject helps neither women nor men. He believes that it should become common knowledge.

Sexuality, and especially women's sexuality, does not receive much attention in medical school. In fact, one female gynecologist approached for this story declined comment, admitting not to know enough about the subject.

Our seemingly *advanced* western culture is badly informed about human sensuality. Medical encyclopedias still do not mention female ejaculation. However, there *is* some information in, *The Complete Guide to Women's Health.*

The quantity of *amrita is* not indicative of how much the woman enjoys her release. Sometimes there does not appear to be any ejaculation at all. "So please, men," I usually say, "don't make it an issue." Some women I've been working with say they experience an intense pleasurable feeling of release and often ejaculate three to nine times or more during one session of sex, each ejaculatory orgasm giving them more pleasure than the previous one.

However, the experience of female ejaculation varies from woman to woman. Some dribble a small amount of fluid while others soak the sheets.

Some women get concerned that they're urinating and they need to be reassured that this is not the case. It is *amrita* they secrete, not urine. In fact *amrita* does not smell or taste like urine.

The G-spot itself has been a subject of controversy since its "discovery" in 1944 by gynecologist Ernst Grafenberg. The 'G' in g-spot stands for Grafenberg, but many women choose to think of it as the goddess spot. In the 1960s, sexologists Masters and Johnson announced that female orgasms occurred primarily through stimulation of the clitoris, not the vagina, where the G-spot is found. The G-spot (Holt, Rinehart, and Winston), a 1982 book by Beverly Whipple, Alice Ladas, and John Perry, refuted this claim and provides ample evidence that the g-spot exists. My colleague, Dr. Gary Schubach, wrote a very enlightening doctoral thesis on the g-spot. You can find it at: http://www.doctorg.com

Some feminists fear that widespread knowledge about female ejaculation will burden women with one more *trick* they must master in bed to feel fully orgasmic. While this is a true concern, I think that withholding knowledge is not the right approach. Educating women about their birthright to full enjoyment of their bodies is a positive approach.

Tantric approaches do not put any pressure on performance for either males or females. In Tantra what is most important is the deep heart to heart connection and caring between the lovers while they experience the pleasure in lovemaking. The goal is connection and deepening intimacy, not performance.

Appendix D

## Tantric Breathing To Achieve Different States of Blissful Arousal

Breath is life. With the first breath we are alive in our bodies as a separate individual and with the last breath we leave our bodies.

We breathe unconsciously on a survival level and Tantra teaches us to breathe consciously to achieve different states of consciousness and excitement or relaxation.

There is a breath:

- To stir up energy,
- To move it around in your own body to places where you need it to open up more
- To send and receive energy back and forth between the lovers
- To start the orgasmic reflex as explained by William Reich
- To intentionally slow down the excitement and refine sexual energy so love making can become a peak experience
- To lift the refined sexual energy to the heart and the head if it becomes too intense to avoid or postpone ejaculation and to deepen love
- To extend the ejaculation duration when and if you choose to ejaculate. Some tantric masters make it last the duration of several long breaths.
- To transform sexual energy into higher spiritual energy
- To go into a meditative union with your lover

- To empower a vision or a deep heart's desire that you have by propelling it into the Universe using the tantrically built-up sexual excitement as a vehicle.

## Appendix E

## Importance of Touch to Build Sexual Charge and Love

In this busy age when we're always pressed for time, people have forgotten what it's like to touch each other just for the pleasure of it. Even if that opportunity arises, the tendency is to get caught up over ejaculatory orgasms. Admittedly, ejaculatory orgasm produces intense pleasure but unless it is built up slowly with conscious touch it is more like a sneeze in the groin, a release of built up tension, than a deeply satisfying experience that *makes love grow* (love *making*).

Unfortunately for many people a sex encounter becomes more like a mutual masturbation session than a real love building experience.

Tantra invites us to take time to thoroughly touch each other to increase arousal across the entire body. Your conscious touch stirs up energy in the form of weak electronic waves that start flowing, continuing to build up until they become larger waves that encompass the entire body. The pleasure waves increase the flow of happy hormones that help open up both the heart and the flow of sexual energy.

When I say conscious I mean that you are not thinking of something else. Your attention is fully on your lover, how they breathe and how they take in your touch. If the receiver holds her or his breath and seems to be into her own thinking, you might ask if they would like a softer or stronger, slower or faster touch, depending on how you are touching them when you see them *disconnect* from what is happening.

This question will get their attention back and you will get a chance to give them the touch they desire. Sometimes we tend to touch how *we* want to be touched instead of tuning in and see how our lover likes it.

Our skin is our biggest organ and needs caring love and attention. But the tantric touch goes deeper than the skin. When you put your intention together with your breath you can feel all the muscles sucking in that attention which goes all the way down to the bones. Yes, bones need love and attention too and that can be done even without having to use deep tissue massage strokes.

Your intention connected with your breath is very powerful and can penetrate quite deep to touch and heal.

Tantric people know that touching a lover does not always have to end in ejaculation. Touch is both sensuous and healing. The most obvious emissaries of love are our arms and the focal points from which love flows are the palms. So when we touch our loved ones we help them heal from any pain or disappointment they might have experienced during the day. They feel that life is worth living just to be touched by you.

Many women tell me that they often cringe when their man starts touching them because they know it will end up in intercourse and they might not be in the mood for it. To prevent this from happening I invite men to set up a just touching time with their beloved. And I recommend that even when she gets all excited you keep your agreement of "just touching" during this time.

Appendix F

**Tantra and Nutrition**

*NOTE: Before starting any diet or exercise regimen consult your health professional. Since we are all different, it is your responsibility to observe reactions and changes in your own body and take the necessary precautions to protect your physical, emotional, and spiritual health.*

Sexual attractiveness is based not on looks but on **radiance** that comes from breathing deeply, taking adequate time for rest, eating the right foods at the right time of day, and from the flexibility of your spine and your legs.

The best healer is the body itself. If you listen to your body, it will tell you how to heal.

Points to pay attention to:

The metabolism tends to be sluggish in the morning and very efficient from 10:00 AM to 2:00 PM. The last meal of the day should be around 7 PM. If you need to eat something later, eat only fruit, which is primarily digested in the intestines. The stomach needs a night of *fast*; that is why we call the first meal of the day a break of the fast or *breakfast*.

Chewing at least 10 times before swallowing is essential for good digestion. The yogis chew 32 times, one for each tooth! Digestion starts in the mouth. Besides, each time you chew you send a message to your brain that you are being nourished and it imagines that you eat more than you actually do. The more you chew, the less food you need to eat. The stomach should be only three quarters full at the end of the meal to allow for best digestion.

When the cells age or become damaged, raw fruits and vegetables will rejuvenate them. They are the best sources for vitamins and minerals and contain water distilled by the sun.

Eat a good balance of *favorable* carbohydrates originating from vegetables and fruits. Avoid white sugar and white flour (refined and bleached, as used in white breads) which have been depleted of all the vitamins and minerals that we need.

Eat protein from nuts, seeds, and, in moderation, eggs and free range chickens, lambs, or cows, as they aren't fed with antibiotics and don't have their movement restricted so that they get fat more quickly. Certain combinations of beans and grains form a chain of complete protein and are broken down by the digestive system into all the essential amino acids necessary. Soybeans are the only beans that have all the essential amino acids.

Eat essential fatty acids; the best source is fish oil such as salmon and olive oil, which help produce the good cholesterol used by the body to produce hormones.

Avoid table salt, which is stripped of potassium and **use sea salt** which is available in most health food stores. Avoid refined sugar because it makes the pancreas secrete abnormally high quantities of insulin and causes the adrenal glands to become depleted. You want highly productive adrenal glands because they produce sex hormones.

Avoid caffeine because it strains your nervous system by making you feel high and then dropping your energy level much lower than it was before. Furthermore it steals calcium from your body.

Because the digestive system performs best when the sun is high in the sky, whether it is sunny or not, the bulk of your eating should take place between 10:00 AM and 2:00 PM. If you are meeting a client for a big dinner the extra energy used for digestion will diminish the energy supply available for sex that night.

If you crave sugar or excessively fatty foods because your body is not quite balanced yet then do it between 10:00 AM and 2:00 PM. After three weeks of following these suggestions you will have lost the desire for sugar or fat-laden foods.

Abdominal breathing helps production of hormones and enzymes needed by the body. It helps your digestion and reduces stress which adversely affects the production of sex hormones.

Both your upper and our lower body need exercise to stay healthy and aid deep breathing and digestion.

Overeating or eating the wrong foods is like putting wet wood on the fire.

You may want to get acquainted with flower essences because they transfer subtle energy that resonates with human feelings and emotions and can help in cases of anxiety and even low self-esteem. The best on the market are the Young Living Essential Oils which I use in my healing practice. Good nutrition cannot be separated from the rest of your life. Rest helps restore all your bodily functions including those of the digestive system. When you feel peaceful within, everything works better. Therefore, before going to bed meditate on your day and come to peace with all the events therein. Ask God to help you be even more aware and loving the next day. Take at least 20 deep abdominal breaths and your sleep will be peaceful and restorative.

Appendix G

**Sexual Dysfunctions**

According to the Journal of the American Medical Association, in 2005 more than 105 million Americans reported struggling with chronic sexual dysfunctions and many of them were not aware that there is help available. Diabetes can be one of the causes of sexual dysfunctions. Prescription medications for depression can also have a negative effect on sexual desire.

There are many causes some of which are related to hormone production, some to blocks in the flow of energy, some to shallow anxious breathing and unhealthy diet, just to mention a few.

The **hormonal production** tends to diminish with age and you could consult a good endocrinologist to check your hormonal production status. Quite a bit of information is available on the internet.

There are also products available that are natural and organic that safely stimulate the body to increase production of the body's natural growth hormones.

What you eat and drink is also important. There are certain simple recommendations you might want to observe most of the time: eat your biggest meal between 12 and 2 PM; eat fish and vegetables often; keep your stomach light at night; drink lots of water during the day. Drinking a little alcohol can help lower inhibitions while drinking too much can inhibit sexuality. For more information, see Appendix F on nutrition.

Printed in the United States
90267LV00005B/16/A